D1314575

LEGAL–ETHICAL CONSIDERATIONS, RESTRICTIONS, AND OBLIGATIONS FOR CLINICIANS WHO TREAT COMMUNICATIVE DISORDERS

LEGAL-ETHICAL CONSIDERATIONS, RESTRICTIONS, AND OBLIGATIONS FOR CLINICIANS WHO TREAT COMMUNICATIVE DISORDERS

Second Edition

By

FRANKLIN H. SILVERMAN, PH.D.

Professor of Speech Pathology
Marquette University, Milwaukee
Clinical Professor of Rehabilitation Medicine
Medical College of Wisconsin, Milwaukee

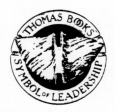

CHARLES C THOMAS • PUBLISHER
Springfield • Illinois • U.S.A.

Published and Distributed Throughout the World by

CHARLES C THOMAS • PUBLISHER
2600 South First Street
Springfield, Illinois 62794-9265

© *1992 by* CHARLES C THOMAS • PUBLISHER
ISBN 0-398-05783-4
Library of Congress Catalog Card Number: 91-36940

With THOMAS BOOKS *careful attention is given to all details of manufacturing
and design. It is the Publisher's desire to present books that are satisfactory as to their
physical qualities and artistic possibilities and appropriate for their particular use.*
THOMAS BOOKS *will be true to those laws of quality that assure a good name
and good will.*

Printed in the United States of America
SC-R-3

Library of Congress Cataloging-in-Publication Data

Silverman, Franklin H., 1933–
    Legal-ethical considerations, restrictions, and obligations for
clinicians who treat communicative disorders / by Franklin H.
Silverman. – 2nd ed.
        p.   cm.
    Rev. ed. of: Legal aspects of speech-language pathology and
audiology. c1983.
    Includes bibliographical references and index.
    ISBN 0-398-05783-4 (cloth)
    1. Speech therapists – Legal status, laws, etc. – United States.
2. Audiologists – Legal status, laws, etc. – United States. 3. Speech
therapists – Professional ethics – United States. 4. Audiologists –
Professional ethics – United States. I. Silverman, Franklin H.,
1933–   Legal aspects of speech-language pathology and audiology
II. Title.
    [DNLM: 1. Audiology – United States – legislation. 2. Ethics,
Medical. 3. Speech-Language Pathology – United States – legislation.
WV 33 S5L]
KF2915.S63S53   1992
344.73'041 – dc20
[347.30441]
DNLM/DLC   91-36940
for Library of Congress   CIP

PREFACE

The clinical functioning of speech-language pathologists and audiologists at any given time is determined not only by their clinical skills and the needs of their clients, but also by *numerous legal-ethical restrictions and obligations.* These come from a number of sources: the Constitution; municipal, county, state, and federal legislation; regulations from state and federal administrative agencies; legal precedents derived from court decisions (i.e., common law); and professional codes of ethics. Speech-language pathologists and audiologists must be aware of the legal-ethical restrictions and obligations they are required by law to consider in their relationships with their clients and their families; with employees, employers, and other professionals; with government agencies; and with all others with whom they interact professionally. Ignorance of the law unfortunately does not protect one from the consequences of violating it!

In this Second Edition of *Legal Aspects of Speech-Language Pathology and Audiology* I have sought to both bring the text up to date and strengthen it. The information on a number of topics has been augmented, particularly professional ethics. The title of the book was changed to reflect this increased emphasis on ethics and to more accurately describe its content.

The book deals with legal-ethical issues that impinge on clinical practice and research in speech-language pathology and audiology. My primary objective is to provide clinicians with the basic information they need to use the law to promote the welfare of those whom they serve professionally without getting themselves into trouble. *This book is not intended to serve as a substitute for legal consultation.* Rather, it is meant to *enhance* such consultation by providing readers with the intuitive understanding of legal concepts that they need to formulate questions that will yield desired information and to interpret the answers given.

Legal-Ethical Considerations, Restrictions, and Obligations for Clinicians who Treat Communicative Disorders is divided into two parts. The first (Chapters 1 and 2) provides basic information about how the law and professional ethics impinge on clinical practice and research and how the legal system functions. The second part (Chapters 3 through 12) provides information about how specific aspects of law and professional ethics both can be applied to promote the welfare of those whom speech-language pathologists and audiologists serve professionally and to protect them from litigation for breach of contract and various torts including malpractice.

The book contains a set of representative release forms (Appendix A); the Nuremberg Code and Declaration of Helsinki, both of which deal with the use of human subjects in research (Appendix B); a listing of legislation relevant to speech-language pathologists and audiologists (Appendix C); selected ethical codes of the American Speech-Language-Hearing Association, 1930–1991 (Appendix D); and a glossary of legal terms.

It is impossible to give credit to the many sources from which the concepts presented in this book have been drawn. The book is the result of years of reading and hundreds of hours of conversation with students and colleagues in the areas of speech-language pathology, audiology, and law. Thus, I cannot credit this or that concept to a specific person, but I can say thank you to all who have helped, particularly my graduate students at Marquette University, whose questions and criticisms through the years have helped me to clarify my own ideas.

Special thanks are due to the American Speech-Language-Hearing Association for giving me the opportunity to serve as the first Wisconsin Coordinator for its Congressional Action Contact Network and to Governor Tommy Thompson of Wisconsin for giving me the opportunity to function as a public official of an administrative agency. It was these experiences that were primarily responsible for my developing and maintaining a strong interest in legal-ethical aspects of our field. Some special thanks also are due to the following persons for their helpful reviews of the book proposal or comments on it: Dr. Arnold E. Aronson, Mayo Clinic; Dr. Daniel Boone, University of Arizona; Dr. Melvin Cohen, Loma Linda University; Dr. Eugene B. Cooper, University of Alabama; Dr. Richard Fowler, University of California; Dr. Sandra C. Holley, Southern Connecticut State University; Attorney Ruth Jakoby, Chevy Chase, Maryland; Attorney Diane Mashie, Washington, D.C.; Dr. Kenneth Moll, University of Iowa; Dr. Thomas J. O'Toole, Montgomery County Public Schools; Dr. Herbert O. Oyer, Ohio State University, and Attorney Philip Padden, Milwaukee, Wisconsin.

Franklin H. Silverman

CONTENTS

LEGAL–ETHICAL CONSIDERATIONS, RESTRICTIONS, AND OBLIGATIONS FOR CLINICIANS WHO TREAT COMMUNICATIVE DISORDERS

Chapter I

RELEVANCE OF LAW AND
PROFESSIONAL ETHICS FOR THE
SPEECH-LANGUAGE PATHOLOGIST
AND AUDIOLOGIST

The clinical functioning of speech-language pathologists and audiologists at any given moment is determined not only by their clinical skills and the needs of their clients but also by numerous *legal-ethical restraints and obligations*. These originate from a number of sources, including the Constitution; municipal, county, state, and federal legislation; regulations from administrative agencies (such as state and federal departments of education); legal precedents derived from court decisions (known as *common law*); and professional codes of ethics (Browne, 1991). Failure to consider these restraints and obligations adequately when functioning clinically can result in such consequences as being fired by one's employer; being sued by a client or a client's family; not being reimbursed by a private or governmental "insurance agency" for services rendered; loss of certification or licensure; and having one's clients not receive services to which they are or should be entitled by law. It is crucial, therefore, that speech-language pathologists and audiologists be aware of the legal-ethical restraints and obligations that they are required by law to consider in their relationships with their clients and their families, employers, employees, other professionals, governmental agencies, and others with whom they interact professionally.

My primary objective in this chapter is to heighten your awareness of the legal-ethical restraints and obligations that influence your functioning as a clinician or clinician-investigator (a clinician who does both clinical work and clinical research — for a discussion of this concept see Chapter 2 of Silverman, 1993). I will attempt to achieve this objective by describing the intersect (i.e., area of overlap) between law, professional ethics, and clinical practice and research (see Figure 1.1). Specific aspects that are dealt with here include the following:

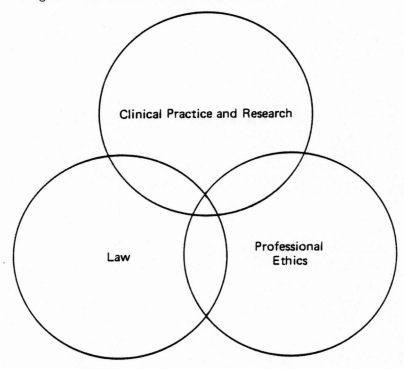

FIGURE 1.1 Intersect between law, professional ethics, and clinical practice and research.

1. The speech-language pathologist and audiologist as a participant in administrative hearings (e.g., those conducted to enforce state and federal school laws)
2. Regulation of speech-language pathology and audiology clinical services by state and federal agencies
3. Litigation for malpractice and other torts
4. The "unwritten" contract inherent in the client-clinician relationship
5. Serving as an expert witness
6. Lobbying for legislation beneficial to the communicatively handicapped and the profession
7. Serving as an advocate for clients
8. Clinical records management
9. Copyright and patent law as it applies to the development and use of clinical and research materials
10. Legal considerations in administering a clinical program
11. Legal considerations in establishing a part-time or full-time private practice

12. Licensure and certification
13. Ethical considerations in clinical practice and research
14. Legal-ethical considerations in the design, conduct, and communication of clinical research
15. Serving as a consultant to a state or federal agency developing regulations affecting the communicatively handicapped or the profession

These, of course, are not the only areas where clinical practice and research, law, and professional ethics overlap. Each is examined here briefly and in more detail elsewhere in the book.

SOME INTERSECTS BETWEEN LAW, PROFESSIONAL ETHICS, AND CLINICAL PRACTICE AND RESEARCH

Participation in Administrative Hearings

As a result of state federal legislation (such as Public Law 94-142) that defines the nature of the services to be provided handicapped children and adults (including the communicatively handicapped), speech-language pathologists and audiologists have become participants in hearings in which the appropriateness of services that have been provided to or recommended for a communicatively handicapped person are being questioned. They have functioned in at least five ways at such hearings. One is as *defendants* (when the appropriateness of the services they have provided or recommended is being questioned). A second is as *ordinary witnesses* (in which they testify about something they saw and/or heard). A third is as *expert witnesses* (in which they are called upon to testify as an "authority" either in court or in a *pretrial deposition* about some aspect(s) of the appropriateness of the services that were provided or recommended). A fourth is as *hearing officers* (in which they function similarly to a judge and hand down a decision). And a fifth is as *advocates* (in which they help the *plaintiff*, the communicatively handicapped person, to obtain the services to which he or she is entitled by law).

Regulation of Services by State and Federal Agencies

The clinical and research activities of speech-language pathologists and audiologists are regulated in many ways by state and federal agencies (see Browne, 1990). State and federal offices of education, for example, regulate the delivery of services to school-age children. The Social Security Administration through Medicare regulates in part the delivery of such services to senior citizens. State licensure boards regulate the practice of both speech-language pathology and audiology. And the National Institutes of Health regulate how human subjects can be used in research. These are only a few of the agencies that regulate speech-language pathology and audiology services and research.

Litigation for Malpractice and Other Torts

A speech-language pathologist or audiologist can be sued by a client, the client's family, a research subject, or another professional for *injuries* or *wrongs* that they claim he or she did while functioning as a clinician or researcher. Civil (as opposed to criminal) injuries or wrongs are known as *torts* (Prosser, 1984). The claimed injury can be to the plaintiff's person or to his or her reputation or feelings. Two examples of a claimed injury to a plaintiff's *person* would be the failure of an audiologist to detect an acoustic neuroma because of using inappropriate testing procedures and the failure of a speech-language pathologist to encourage a patient who had a hoarse voice because of carcinoma to be examined by a laryngologist before beginning voice therapy with him or her. The *negligence* tort that the plaintiff probably would claim had occurred in both instances would be *malpractice*. A claimed injury to the *reputation* or *feelings* of a plaintiff who is a professional could occur if a speech-language pathologist or audiologist *orally* indicated to potential clients that the professional was unethical or incompetent (tort of *slander*). If the reference was made in *writing,* the tort would be that of *libel.*

The "Unwritten" Contract Inherent in the Client-Clinician Relationship

The relationship between client and clinician is governed, in part, by *contract law* (Corbin, 1991). When a clinician offers to provide therapy for a client and the client (or someone legally responsible for him or her) accepts the offer, a contract may be formed between them. Contracts need not be written to be legally enforceable. Problems develop when the terms of the contract—that is, the obligations that both parties assume under it—are not fully understood by both parties. A client, for example, may assume that by offering therapy a clinician is indicating an ability to cure a particular disorder. If the clinician fails to cure it, the client may regard the contract as having been *breached* and refuse to pay for some or all of the clinician's services or lodge a complaint against him or her with the state licensing board or the American Speech-Language-Hearing Association (A.S.H.A.). A knowledge of contract law can help to prevent such misunderstandings.

Serving as an Expert Witness

Speech-language pathologists and audiologists are asked to testify as experts in their fields in both federal and state courts and administrative hearings (such as those associated with implementation of P.L. 94-142 which mandates that school districts meet the educational needs of all handicapped children for whom they are responsible). They may serve in this role at the request of either the plaintiff or defendant in a case that is to be heard by a court or of any of the parties involved in an administrative hearing. A speech-language pathologist, for example, may be asked to testify about the competency of an aphasic to continue to manage his or her financial affairs; an audiologist may be asked to testify about the status of a plaintiff's hearing in a worker's compensation case.

Lobbying for Legislation Beneficial to the Communicatively Handicapped and the Profession

Since the providing of clinical services and the conduct of research is regulated by both state and federal legislation, speech-language pathologists and audiologists should have some interest in encouraging legislators at both state and federal levels to support bills that benefit the communicatively handicapped and the profession and to amend and not support bills that could be detrimental to either or both. They can do this by informing their representatives specifically why they feel it would be in society's best interest if a particular bill were supported, amended, or voted down. By assuming this responsibility they increase the probability that their legislators will consider the issues they have raised when deciding how to vote on a bill. Most senators and representatives appreciate such lobbying because it helps them cast more informed votes. Some speech-language pathologists and audiologists devote considerable time to lobbying through participation in the Congressional Action Contact Network of the American Speech-Language-Hearing Association (Dowling, 1973) and those of some state speech, language, and hearing associations that have been modeled after it.

Serving as an Advocate for Clients

Speech-language pathologists have a responsibility to ensure that their clients receive the services to which they are entitled by law. To assume this responsibility they must be aware of statutes (such as P.L. 94-142), administrative agency regulations (such as those *promulgated* by state Departments of Public Instruction), and court decisions dealing with both of these that could facilitate the delivery of services to their clients, for example, by providing funding. In some cases they can play this advocacy role merely by making a client or a client's family aware of them. In other cases speech-language pathologists and audiologists serve as intermediaries between the client or family and the agency from whom assistance is being sought by providing the agency with information about the client or indicating to an agency why the client appears to be entitled to certain services. Speech-language pathologists and audiologists may also have to serve as advocates for reasons unrelated to their client's communicative behaviors. A speech-language pathologist employed in a school, for example, may have to assume an advocacy role for a client who appears to be a "battered child" (O'Toole, 1974).

Clinical Records Management

Speech-language pathologists and audiologists, regardless of the setting in which they work, are required to maintain records on their clients. Management of such records has legal-ethical considerations. The confidentiality of the information in them must be maintained, and at the same time it must be possible to release specific information in them to other professionals or agencies when a client or client's family request that it be done. Also, they must be maintained in such a manner that the client's or his or her family's freedom of access to them (which is mandated by law) is unlikely to be detrimental to either client or clinician. Another important consideration concerns *subpoena* procedures: what must be released under certain circumstances, the rights of the client in such circumstances, and monitoring the content of record entries with a view to the possibility of subpoena.

Copyright and Patent Law

Speech-language pathologists and audiologists are both consumers and producers of copyrighted and patented materials and apparatus. There are legal restrictions on how such materials and apparatus can be utilized and reproduced for clinical, educational, and research purposes. Some such restrictions are imposed by the Copyright Act of 1976. Under this act, all materials developed by or for clinicians are *automatically* protected by copyright, regardless of whether they have been distributed commercially or have been formally copyrighted and regardless of whether they are printed or on computer disks, compact disks (CDs) audiotapes, or videotapes (see Chickering & Hartman, 1987).

Administering Clinical Programs

Speech-language pathologists and audiologists (whether in private practice or working in a school, hospital, or other clinical setting) are often called on to function as administrators, a role with legal-ethical aspects. When hiring employees (at both professional and clerical levels), for example, they must comply with federal regulations prohibiting discrimination against women, minorities, and the handicapped. They also must be in compliance with federal regulations when developing and managing a clinical record system. In addition, they must be aware of ethical considerations when deciding how to make the public aware of their clinical services. These are a only a few of the legal-ethical restrictions and obligations that administrators of clinical programs must consider.

Establishing a Private Practice

There are a number of legal-ethical considerations when establishing a part-time or full-time private practice, many of which were mentioned in the preceding section on administering a clinical program. In addition, since a private practice is a *small business*, municipal, state, and federal regulations for establishing and operating such businesses must be followed. A legal structure for the practice must be selected — should it be set up as a proprietorship, partnership, or corporation? (Some professionals in private practice incorporate in order to reduce their personal financial liability if they should be unsuccessful.) Also, a bookkeeping system that is adequate for tax and other purposes must be established.

Licensure and Certification

Legal-ethical restrictions on clinical practice in speech-language pathology and audiology are imposed by state licensure laws and American Speech-Language-Hearing Association certification. Every state, through a department that oversees public instruction, credentials speech-language pathologists who want to work in its public schools. Many states license speech-language pathologists and audiologists who do not work in the schools. The requirements for such licenses, incidentally, tend to be quite similar to those for the Certificates of Clinical Competence in Speech-Language Pathology and Audiology awarded by the American Speech-Language-Hearing Association.

Ethical Considerations in Clinical Practice and Research

Speech-language pathologists and audiologists, like the members of all professions, are required to function in a manner consistent with a code (or codes) of professional ethics and a "higher" ethical code, that of their society. The American Speech-Language-Hearing Association (Code of Ethics of the American Speech-Language-Hearing Association, 1991) and some state speech, language, and hearing associations have such codes. These codes impose both restrictions and obligations on clinical practice in speech-language pathology and audiology. For example, they both restrict the types of disorders practitioners can treat (e.g., persons certified in audiology cannot treat stuttering unless they are also certified in speech-language pathology) and oblige them to refer clients to other professionals (physicians, dentists, psychologists, other speech-language pathologists or audiologists, etc.) when such referrals would appear to be in their best interest. The professional activities of practitioners also are influenced by "higher" ethical codes. One such code that would influence their functioning in the United States is *Judeo-Christian ethics.* An aspect of this code that is relevant clinically is referred to in the bioethics literature as the *ethics of manipulation* (Haring, 1975). This deals with ethical considerations when planning how to manipulate or control the behavior of a client.

Legal Considerations in Clinical Research

A number of legal-ethical restrictions and obligations must be considered in the design, conduct, and communication of clinical research. Most are intended to protect the person, reputation, and feelings of research subjects. Investigators, for example, must be able to document that they have obtained the *informed consent* of the persons who are serving as subjects in their studies (Freund, 1970). For their consent to be *informed,* subjects must be made aware of any possible adverse effects they could experience as a result of participation in the research. Investigators are also required to protect subjects from harm to their reputations and feelings when reporting the results of their research, either keeping the identities of subjects unrecognizable or obtaining an appropriate release from them. Obtaining a release is particularly important when still photographs, motion pictures, audiotapes, or videotapes may be used as a part of the presentation of the research findings. (A form that can be used for this purpose is included in Appendix A.)

Serving as a Consultant to a State or Federal Agency

Speech-language pathologists and audiologists have served as consultants to state or federal agencies while they were developing regulations affecting the communicatively handicapped or the profession. One of the main ways they have done so is as members of advisory councils. Such councils, for example, have been established by state agencies that license speech-language pathologists and audiologists. They also have been established by those that are responsible for implementing provisions of particular federal laws—for example, the Telecommunications Relay Service provision of the Americans with Disabilities Act of 1990. They usually are appointed to such councils by the governor and while serving on them function as *public officials*.

Chapter II

OUR LEGAL SYSTEM:
AN OVERVIEW OF
PROFESSIONALLY RELEVANT ASPECTS

In the preceding chapter we briefly considered some of the impacts our legal system has on clinical practice and research in speech-language pathology and audiology. Before exploring such impacts in greater depth, we shall consider the overall structure of our legal system, particularly those aspects that are important for understanding the intersect between law and clinical practice and research (see Figure 1.1).

We will begin by defining law through a consideration of its impacts on interpersonal relationships. Our entire system of law can be viewed as being motivated by a desire to control or regulate aspects of the various types of interpersonal relationships in which people participate in our society.

Next, we will consider sources from which laws that seek to influence aspects of our interpersonal relationships arise. Among those that will be dealt with are courts (common law), legislatures (federal, state, and municipal statutes), and professional organizations (e.g., regulations from the American Speech-Language-Hearing Association concerning clinical certification). While professional organizations (such as A.S.H.A.) are not generally regarded as sources of laws, they tend to function in ways that make them de facto lawmaking bodies.

Next, the internal structure of our legal system will be described, including the types, or categories, of law contained in it. This will include a discussion of the distinctions among (1) criminal, administrative, and civil law, (2) substantive and procedural law, and (3) common law and legislative statutes. Finally, we will consider the mechanisms used for *enforcing* laws, with particular emphasis on the civil suit and administrative hearing.

WHAT ARE LAWS?

Laws are rules courts will enforce that are intended to govern our interpersonal relationships. They place *restrictions* and *obligations* on our relationships with others. Failure to obey them is ordinarily *supposed* to result in some sort of penalty.

Laws, viewed as rules intended for governing interpersonal relationships, vary on several dimensions (aside from specific content) including:

1. **The number of persons to which they are applicable.** Regulations from the Wisconsin Department of Public Instruction concerning maximum and minimum sizes for public school speech-language pathologists' caseloads are applicable to fewer persons than regulations arising from a federal statute such as Public Law 94-142 (see Appendix C).

2. **Their relative strength.** Some laws are viewed as stronger than others in the sense that they have *precedence* over them. If two laws of unequal strength are applicable to a specific situation, the stronger usually will prevail. If, for example, the regulations from a state department of public instruction indicated that school districts could be reimbursed for speech-language pathology services only for children whose communicative disorder is "educationally significant" and if a federal statute indicated that the criterion of educational significance could not be used to deny funding for such services, the federal statute would probably prevail because federal statutes usually have precedence over state statutes when both apply to the same situation.

3. **Their source.** The rules or laws that regulate our interpersonal relationships as speech-language pathologists or audiologists arise from a number of sources, including municipal, state, and federal legislation; state and federal constitutions; precedents from court decisions; regulations from state and federal administrative agencies; professional codes of ethics (such as that of the American Speech-Language-Hearing Association); and regulations established by employers. While an employer's regulations are usually not thought of as "laws," they function as such in that one is expected to obey them or pay a penalty (e.g., receive a reprimand or be fired). Also, they are implicitly recognized as laws by the courts since they must be consistent with municipal, state, and federal laws. If, for example, an employer made a regulation that members of certain minority groups could not be hired, this regulation probably would be declared illegal by the courts (if they were asked to rule on it) because state and federal legislation, which has precedence

over employers' regulations, prohibits discrimination in hiring. Sources of law are considered in greater depth elsewhere in this chapter.

4. **Their duration.** Some laws remain in effect only for a specified period of time; others remain in effect until some action is taken to change or terminate them. As a result of *sunset laws,* some state licensure boards for speech-language pathologists and audiologists terminate after a specific number of years unless the legislation that created them is reenacted by the legislature (Downey, 1979).

5. **Their degree of specificity.** The restrictions and obligations mandated by some laws are presented at a lower level of abstraction (Johnson, 1946) then they are for others. They are specified in greater detail. The two quotations that follow illustrate this dimension. They are from the laws of two states pertaining to minimum requirements for facilities for providing speech, language, and hearing therapy in the public schools.

> The school system shall provide a classroom of suitable size, in a distraction free area as required by the type of program or services to be established, with appropriate furniture, materials, supplies and equipment to meet the needs of the class or individual children to be served.
>
> For speech, language, and hearing therapy services, a quiet, adequately lighted and ventilated room with an electrical outlet must be provided at each center for the exclusive use of the speech, language, and hearing therapist, during the times scheduled at the center. The space at each center must have one table with five medium size chairs, one teacher's chair, one bulletin board, one permanent or portable chalkboard, and one large mirror mounted so that the therapist and student may sit before it. (Both quotations are from the *Digest of State Laws and Regulations for School Language, Speech, and Hearing Programs,* 1973.)

Obviously, the degree of specificity is greater (and the level of abstraction is lower) for the second than it is for the first.

6. **The probability that they will be obeyed.** Some laws (regulations) are more likely to be obeyed than are others. A law may not be obeyed because at least some of the restrictions or obligations it imposes are contrary to the desires of the majority of the people to whom it applies (e.g., the "prohibition" amendment to the Constitution and the 55 mile an hour speed limit). Or a law may not be obeyed because it is viewed as inconsistent with natural law—that is, what one considers "right" or "fair." (Some men left the country to avoid the draft during the Vietnam War because they considered the war to be "wrong.") Finally, some people may not obey a law because the restrictions or obligations imposed

by it are contrary to their desires, and they are willing to risk receiving a penalty for not obeying it (e.g., some people do not report *all* their income to the I.R.S.).

WHY ARE LAWS OBEYED?

Our willingness (or lack of willingness) to obey the laws that make up our legal system can be rationalized, or explained, by certain philosophies (or principles) in which we believe. Representative ones are summarized in Figure 2.1. We utilize such philosophies (whether or not we are consciously aware of doing so) when deciding the extent to which we are willing to accept particular restrictions and obligations in our interpersonal relationships.

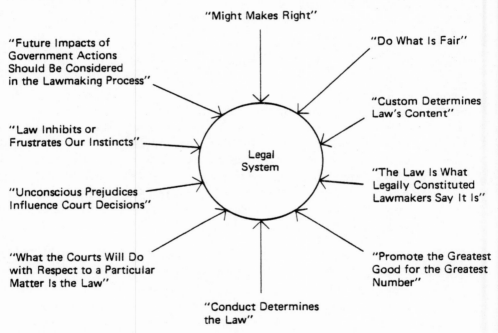

FIGURE 2.1 Some philosophies that have influenced and are influencing our legal system.

The philosophies included in Figure 2.1, which are those that appear to exert the greatest influence on our behavior, will be described briefly. (For further information about them see Fisher, 1977, pp. 2–25, which was the primary source for this discussion.)

"Might Makes Right"

This philosophy suggests that we may accept restrictions and obligations because we view the source requesting us to do so as stronger than ourselves. Some clinicians (particularly student clinicians) accept supervisors' recommendations on this basis.

"Do What is Fair"

This philosophy suggests that we have an obligation in our interpersonal relationships to what is "right," "fair," "just," and "ethical." It further suggests that we are obliged to not do what is "wrong," "unfair," "unjust," and "unethical" *even if doing so is required by law.* This philosophy, which is known as *natural law,* is an aspect of our Judeo-Christian tradition. It assumes the existence of certain values that are so self-evident (perhaps God-given) that if laws are in conflict with them they should not be obeyed. When we use our *conscience* as a guide for determining our behavior, we are functioning on the basis of natural law. Violating such law results in *guilt* feelings. Natural law, of course, is the source of much of our law. Its main limitation is the lack of universal agreement about what behavior is "right," "fair," "just," and "ethical." Affirmative action programs in hiring for women and minorities illustrate this problem. By behaving in a manner that probably would be viewed as "fair" by one segment of the population (i.e., giving women and minorities preferential treatment in hiring), one would be behaving in a manner that probably would be viewed as "unfair" by another—those who lose jobs to women and minority group members who they regard as being less qualified than themselves.

Much of our functioning as speech-language pathologists and audiologists is motivated by a desire to do what is *fair.* For example, we believe that our services should be available to any communicatively handicapped person who is likely to profit from them and that it would be *unfair* for such a person to be deprived of them because of an inability to pay. We feel it is only *fair* in such instances that a government agency or other third party pay for the required services.

"Custom Determines Law's Content"

This philosophy suggests that our interpersonal relationships are regulated, in part, by custom or tradition. What has been regarded as acceptable (lawful) behavior is likely to continue to be regarded as such and vice versa. An employer may expect a clinician to function in a certain manner (e.g., maintain a caseload of a particular size or schedule his or her clients in a particular way) because it has been the custom at that institution for clinicians to do so. What is required by custom can be either "good" or "bad," "fair" or "unfair."

Rules (laws) that are not consistent with tradition are likely to be disobeyed. A classic example of this phenomenon was public reaction to the Eighteenth Amendment to the United States Constitution which prohibited the manufacture and sale of intoxicating liquors for human consumption. This law was unenforceable and had to be repealed by the Twenty-First Amendment.

Clinicians who are prohibited from treating clients they have traditionally been allowed to treat may continue to treat them. During 1970s, for example, school clinicians in one state were told by their department of public instruction to exclude from their caseloads children who had communicative disorders that were not "educationally significant," such as those having only a single articulation error (e.g., a w/r substitution). Nevertheless many continued to include some of them in their caseloads.

"The Law is What Legally Constituted Lawmakers Say it is"

The philosophies that we have discussed — the will of the stronger, the concept of fairness, and accepted custom — are not what most persons regard as the content of law. Most people view our legal system as consisting of *rules* (e.g., constitutions, statutes, ordinances, case law made by judges, and administrative regulations) that are promulgated by an individual or group (e.g., a legislature, court, administrative agency, professional organization, or employer) who is (1) legally authorized to promulgate such rules and (2) has made them in the manner indicated by a constitution (or other document setting forth rule-making procedures) that members of the group have accepted as binding on them. The act of accepting membership in a group, whether citizenship in a country, membership in an organization, or employment in an institution, implies a willingness to accept both the rules and rule-making procedures of that group. Of course, one is free to attempt to change a rule, but one is obligated to do it by means of the procedures outlined in the group's constitution (or other document that specifies rule-changing procedures). This view of law, which is referred to as *positive law* or *analytical positivism*, is the main philosophical foundation of the United States legal system.

Rules (laws) promulgated by a group who accept this philosophy as the foundation of their legal system are supposed to be accepted by the members of the group *regardless of whether these rules are viewed by them as fair or unfair, desirable or undesirable, and consistent with tradition or not consistent with tradition.* So long as they were made in the appropriate manner and are being promulgated by the appropriate person or persons, the members of the group are expected to obey them. Violation of such a rule ordinarily is supposed to result in sanctions. Possible sanctions can include a fine, a jail sentence, or expulsion from the group. Speech-language pathologists and audiologists who are found to be functioning clinically in a manner not consistent with the Code of Ethics of the American Speech-Language-Hearing Association (and thus violating one or more of its rules) can be expelled from the organization (see Actions of the Ethical Practice Board, 1986, 1988, 1989a, 1989b, 1991).

"Promote the Greatest Good for the Greatest Number"

This philosophy, which is known as *utilitarianism*, suggest that legislatures (and other law makers) should attempt to promote the greatest good for the greatest number of persons by making appropriate laws (regulations). The tendency for groups to base decisions on a majority vote can be viewed as an implicit recognition of this philosophy. Its main limitation is that it can be used to justify ignoring the rights of minorities.

"Conduct Determines the Law"

This philosophy suggests that conduct and law can be interrelated in such a manner that the former will influence the latter. How people behave when confronted by a specific set of circumstances can determine what the law says about how people should behave when confronted by that set of circumstances. The probability that a law will be obeyed is partially a function of how consistent it is with conduct *at the time attempts are made to enforce it.* The 55 mile an hour speed limit was increased to 65 miles an hour on some highways because it was more consistent with conduct.

"What the Courts Will Do with Respect to a Particular Matter is the Law"

This philosophy, known as *functionalism*, suggests that the decision the courts are most likely to make in a particular situation can be regarded as the law in that situation. The emphasis here is on judge-made, or common, law. From this perspective, a court decision must be made on a specific legal problem before one can know what the law is. One implication of this philosophy is that a person can do something that is not prohibited by any legislation or regulations, and that action can be regarded as unlawful at some future date if a court is asked to rule on it. Unfortunately, we are frequently confronted by matters for which the law is unclear and will only become clear when the courts have handed down a decision. The best we can do when confronted by such a situation is to try to predict what the courts will do. Consultation with a lawyer is usually necessary to make such a prediction knowledgeably.

Uncertainty about what the law is can arise when federal legislation is developed to regulate an area formerly regulated by state legislation. If aspects of the existing state statute(s) differ from the federal one, which should be obeyed? It could be argued that the federal one should be obeyed because it is *stronger* than (i.e., has precedence over) the state one. It might also be possible to argue that the federal law merely sets *minimum* standards and that the state law, because it sets *tougher* standards, should be the applicable one. It might not be clear, however, which sets tougher standards. In such a situation the courts would have to decide what is the law.

"Unconscious Prejudices Influence Court Decisions"

The philosophies considered thus far have dealt with the law as if its interpretation were independent of the person or persons interpreting it. They implicitly assume that the motivations and prejudices of law-makers and interpreters (e.g., judges and juries) do not influence the content of law and how it is interpreted and applied. In other words, they seem to assume that "justice is blind." Such an assumption is counterintuitive. There is a philosophy known as *realism* that does take such factors into consideration when defining law. Those who accept this philosophy view the law *as we know it* as involving an interaction between the observer and the observed (Johnson, 1946). The observers' (e.g., judges and juries) attitudes are regarded as influencing how they inter-pret the observed (the law). Fisher has noted:

> In deciding cases it was perceived that unconscious prejudices judges held respecting the likelihood of someone's having committed a crime, the judge's view of the good or evil that motivated a defendant, and the basic likes and dislikes of the judge, affect a decision more than applicable rules. Realists believe that superficialities such as dress, skin color, age, occupation, and vocabulary are unacknowledged factors entering into the calculus determinative of criminal guilt or innocence or civil liability or

nonliability. Juries' prejudices similarly influence their verdicts quite apart from objective evidence (Fisher, 1977, p. 19).

Such extraneous factors, of course, enter into the administration (enforcement) of rules at all levels. A given infraction is apt to be reacted to, in part, on the basis of the perceived status of the person breaking the rule. The higher the rule breaker's perceived status, the weaker the penalty is apt to be. An administrator who breaks a rule (e.g., arriving at work late) is apt to be dealt with less severely by an employer than an unskilled worker who breaks the same rule.

"Law Inhibits or Frustrates Our Instincts"

We have viewed law thus far from the perspective of its impact on overt behavior. We have considered how laws can influence interpersonal relationships by imposing restrictions and obligations on our functioning in such relationships. Law can also be viewed from the perspective of its impacts on our *covert*, or internal physiological, functioning. It can influence our emotional status by frustrating instincts. How can law-related frustration affect our emotional functioning? As Fisher has noted:

> There are obvious individual costs of law's being a frustration mechanism: ulcers, high blood pressure, heart attacks, neuroses, and other psychological problems are to some extent manifestations of frustration. Rather than shout a slanderous remark at another or punch someone in the nose and incur legal liability, a civilized person controls his (or her) frustrations and instead risks ulcers and the other health hazards noted above (Fisher, 1977, p. 22).

Of course, it is reasonable to assume that a society in which there is no law (i.e., anarchy) also would be likely to have a detrimental impact on our emotional status and, thereby, on our physiological functioning.

"Future Impacts of Government Actions Should be Considered in the Lawmaking Process"

The philosophies described thus far have had a significant impact on our legal system since its beginnings. This final one, which is of relatively recent origin, pertains to decision making in the lawmaking process. It attempts to introduce into this process safeguards that should increase the probability that lawmakers will think before they leap (Fisher, 1977). Its application forces them to attempt to predict the probable overall impact (both desirable and undesirable consequences) of alternative courses of action that could be used for solving a particular problem. It is hoped that so doing will reduce the odds that the course of action selected for solving a particular problem will create more problems than it eliminates.

FROM WHAT SOURCES DO OUR LAWS ORIGINATE?

In the first two sections of this chapter we attempted to define the term *law* and to describe some of the philosophies that have influenced the laws that make up our legal system. In this section we shall describe some of the origins of the laws (rules, regulations, etc.) that seek to influence aspects of our interpersonal relationships. We shall include courts, legislatures, administrative agencies, and professional organizations. Although not the only sources from which the laws we are expected to obey arise, they are responsible for promulgating the majority of them.

The Courts

One of the main components of our legal system are decisions handed down by judges. These are ordinarily referred to as *common law;* and through application of the doctrine of *stare decisis*, they serve as precedents for future court decisions. In some courts when a case is decided the judge writes a report to be published that summarizes the "facts" of the case indicating his or her decision and the reasons for reaching it (or at least the reasons that the judge is willing to acknowledge).

The process through which court opinions are transformed into law by application of the doctrine of *stare decisis* can be summarized as follows:

> Given a determination of the facts in a dispute, *assuming no controlling law* [italics mine], a court decides the case on the basis of what it believes the law is or should be. In determining what the law is or should be, it looks first to prior decisions resolving similar or analogous disputes and seeks to apply the underlying rules or principles that appear to have been established by those decisions. If the facts presented to the court include the same significant facts as appeared in a previously decided case, without additional facts that could be regarded as significant, the court frequently will bow to the authority of the decision in the prior case and follow it, reaching the same result in the pending case.... If no prior decided case presented the same significant facts, the court will consider whether any prior decided case nevertheless has sufficient elements in common with the pending dispute to require or justify application of

a rule or principle derivable from or underlying the decision in such a prior case (Rombauer, 1978, p. 5).

The phrase "assuming no controlling written law" was italicized to highlight the fact that if there is a controlling written law that applies to the facts in a case, the doctrine of *stare decisis* ordinarily will not be applied. Thus, this doctrine functions to fill gaps in our legal system, the gaps arising from the absence of written law (e.g., statutes).

The opinions of some courts carry more weight as legal precedent than those of others. Each state and territory (e.g., Guam and Puerto Rico) has a court system as has the federal government. While the state and territorial court systems are independent of each other, each interfaces with the federal court system. The opinions of the highest court in each state and territory can be appealed to the United States Supreme Court. The hierarchical organization of state and federal court systems is illustrated in Figure 2.2. Note that both systems contain two types of courts: trial and appellate.

Trial courts are at the low (entrance) level of the hierarchy in both state and federal systems (see Figure 2.2). They are the first courts to try, consider, or become involved with any civil or criminal case. Their functioning can be summarized as follows:

> A trial court hears and decides controversies by determining facts and applying appropriate rules. The opposing parties to a dispute argue their positions by presenting arguments on the law and evidence on the facts in the form of documents and testimony before witnesses. This is done before a single judge sometimes in the presence of a jury. In a trial without a jury, the judge controls the entire trial and determines the outcome. In a trial with a jury, the decision-making functions are divided between the judge and the jury. A safeguard of checks and balances in the legal process is achieved this division of responsibility: The judge determines the correct law to be applied and decides the questions of law; the jury decides what the facts are and applies to those facts the law as stated by the judge. The judge controls the entire litigation. His [or her] actions and statements are often persuasive in the decision-making process of the jury (Grilliot, 1979, pp. 43, 45).

Appellate courts review the decisions of trial courts when they are requested to do so. Such a request, or appeal, may be made by either the defendant or plaintiff in a civil action if either feels that the court that tried the case did not interpret and/or apply the law appropriately (i.e., if he or she feels that the court reached a decision that was not consistent

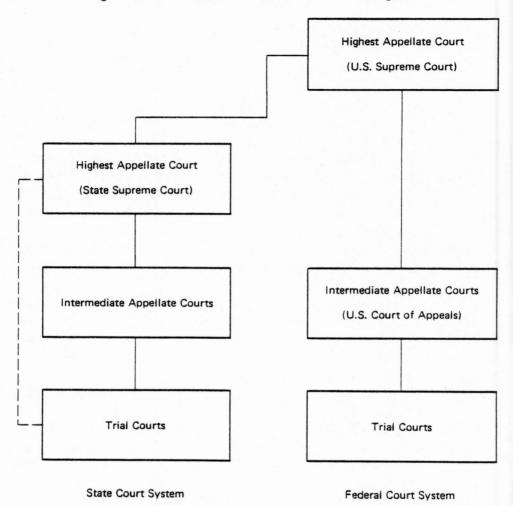

FIGURE 2.2 Hierarchy of courts in state and federal court systems.

with the law or conducted itself in a manner that was not consistent with the law). If an appellate court feels that the decision of a trial court is not legally justifiable, it can nullify (or reverse) it. The functioning of an appellate court can be summarized as follows:

An appellate court's power is confined to the review of errors committed in the court below in the case which is brought up in the appeal. It reviews the proceedings of the trial court to ascertain whether it acted in accordance with the law. The appellate court reaches its decision by using only the record of the proceedings in the lower court, the written briefs filed by both parties to the appeal, and the parties' oral arguments given before the appellate judges. . . . The court bases its decision solely on the theories argued and evidence presented in the lower court; no new arguments or proof are admissible. There are no witnesses or jury at the appellate level. The appellate court does not retry the facts of the case (Grilliot, 1979, p. 46).

Both state and federal systems contain several types of trial and appellate courts. These are indicated for a "typical" state court system in Figure 2.3, which is an elaboration of the left half of Figure 2.2. In this system there are six types of trial courts—justice of the peace, domestic relations, probate, county, municipal, and superior courts—and two types of appellate courts—intermediate and state supreme. Some states have fewer types of trial courts in their systems and others have more, including separate juvenile courts, or small-claims courts, or both. The same also is true for the appellate court component of state systems. Some have a single appellate court, the state supreme court; others have both intermediate appellate courts and a state supreme court. (This distinction between state systems is indicated in Figure 2.2 by the presence of two paths from a state trial court to a state supreme court.) In a state system that contains intermediate appellate courts, trial court decisions initially would usually be appealed to one of these rather than to the state supreme court.

The types of trial and appellate courts in the federal system are shown graphically in Figure 2.4 (which is an elaboration of the right half of Figure 2.2). In this system as diagramed, there are five types of trial courts (i.e., customs, claims, administrative agency, U.S. district with federal and local jurisdiction, and U.S. district with federal jurisdiction only) and three types of appellate courts (i.e., customs and patent appeals, U.S. courts of appeals, and the U.S. Supreme court).

The specific type of trial court that an attorney for a plaintiff would regard as most appropriate for a specific *civil action* would be determined by the answers to a series of questions, including the following:

1. Do both the plaintiff and defendant reside in the same state? If they do, then a trial court in either the state or federal system may be possible. If they do not, then a trial court in the federal system usually would be selected (unless, of course, the defendant was willing to accept the jurisdiction of the plaintiff's state court).
2. How much money is the plaintiff seeking from the defendant? Ordinarily if the amount is relatively small (e.g., less than 50,000) and there is no specific reason why the case would have to be tried in the federal system (e.g., the defendant residing in a different state) the case will be tried in the plaintiff's state system.
3. What is the subject matter of the suit? Some trial courts have *limited*

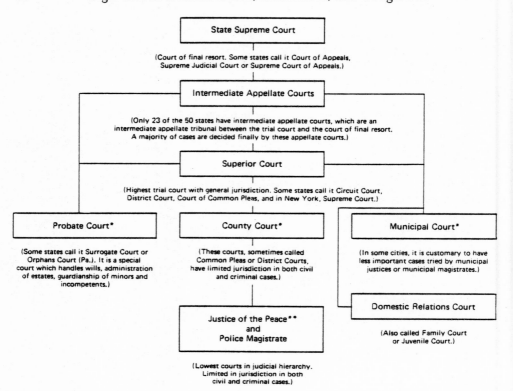

FIGURE 2.3 Hierarchy of courts in a "typical" state system. (Adapted and used with permission from INTRODUCTION TO THE LEGAL SYSTEM, Second Edition by Bruce D. Fisher. Copyright 1977 by West Publishing Company. All rights reserved.)

jurisdiction, which means they can only try cases that deal with a particular subject matter (e.g., juveniles). Others have *general jurisdiction*. They are authorized to handle any subject matter.

4. Does the suit involve a question of violation of a federal statute (or statutes)? Examples would be cases claiming violations in the area of civil rights or of copyrights. Federal courts usually have jurisdiction in such cases, regardless of the amount of money involved.

5. Which court, of those that will accept jurisdiction, is most likely to decide in favor of the client? The attorney for the plaintiff may find, based on a court's (or judge's) record of decisions in similar cases that it may or may not be advantageous for the case to be tried in that court (or by that judge). Given a choice, lawyers will select the court (or judge) most likely to decide for their clients.

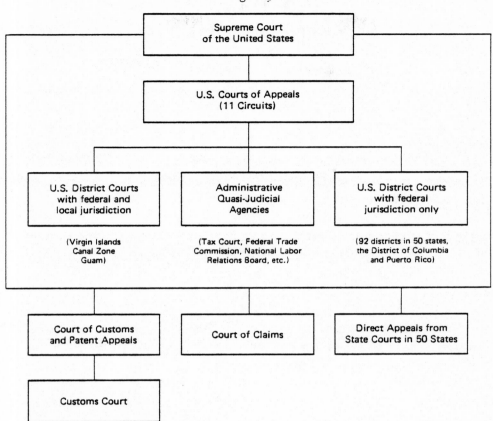

FIGURE 2.4 Hierarchy of courts in the federal system. (Adapted and used with permission from INTRODUCTION TO THE LEGAL SYSTEM, Second Edition by Bruce D. Fisher. Copyright 1977 by West Publishing Company. All rights reserved.)

The court (or judge) selected by the plaintiff in a civil action will not usually be changed unless the defendant can show that there is very good reason for doing so.

Legislatures

The most obvious sources from which laws originate are municipal, state, and federal legislatures. A legislature is "a body of public officials who collectively have the authority to make generalized law for future application" (Grilliot, 1979, p. 550). Those who serve as members of legislatures in almost all instances are elected to serve in this capacity for a specified period of time by geographically defined groups of people whose interests they are supposed to represent. Such a geographically defined group (or *constituency*) could consist of persons who live in a particular section of a large city or in one of several adjacent smaller cities. Presumably, a legislator's constituents can get him or her to represent their interests by indicating through face-to-face contact, a telephone call, a letter, or a telegram how they feel about particular legislation. Even a relatively small number of letters or telegrams from constituents indicating why they believe their legislators should vote in a particular way on a particular *bill* can significantly affect the outcome of the vote on that bill (see Chapter 12). The legislative branch of a municipal (local) government is variously referred to by such terms as the city council, the board of aldermen, or the common council. The legislative branch of state government is referred to as the state legislature and that of the federal government as the United States Congress.

Both state and federal legislatures consist of two branches, with the exception of Nebraska, which has a unicameral legislature. The most prestigious of the two, known as the *senate*, usually has fewer members than the other, which is known as the *house of representatives* or *state assembly*. Thus, senators tend to represent a larger constituency than do members of the house of representatives.

The authority for the United States Congress to exercise its lawmaking function is contained in Article 1 of the United States Constitution. In Section 18 of this article it states that Congress shall have the power "To make all laws which shall be necessary and proper for carrying into Execution . . . all . . . powers vested by this Constitution of the Government of the United States, or any department or office thereof." The Constitution thus gives Congress broad authority for making laws. It also places limits on this lawmaking ability. The framers (and amenders) of the Constitution prohibited Congress from making certain types of laws to protect what they regarded as inalienable rights of United States citizens. Included here are *ex post facto laws* "which make a crime of an act which when committed was not a crime" (Black, 1968, p. 662). A hypothetical example of the application of an *ex post facto* law would be a speech-language pathologist or audiologist being charged with violating the Code of Ethics of the American Speech-Language-Hearing Association because he or she violated a part of the Code *that was not a part of it* at the time that he or she did so. These restrictions on the lawmaking function of Congress also include limitations on its power to pass laws restricting religion, speech, the press, and the right to assemble peaceably (First Amendment) and depriving people of life, liberty, or property without *due process of law* (Fifth Amendment).

The authority for state legislatures to exercise their lawmaking functions "to preserve the public health, safety, morals, and welfare" (Grilliot, 1979, p. 338) existed prior to the framing of the United States Constitution and hence was not derived from it. The legislatures of the thirteen colonies had assumed this function because of their belief in the right of every *sovereignty* (i.e., governmental unit) to pass laws for its internal regulation. This right was accepted without reservation by the framers of the Constitution, although they did set limits on the types of subject matter about which state legislatures could pass laws (see Article 1, Section 10, of the Constitution). The Tenth Amendment states that "The powers not delegated to the United States by the Constitution, nor prohibited to it by the States, are reserved to the States respectively, or to the people." Municipal governmental units derive authority for their lawmaking functions on a similar basis—that is, the right of a governmental unit to pass laws for its internal regulation within limits set by state and federal constitutions.

The process by which proposed laws (*bills*) are transformed by a legislature into laws (*statutes*) consists of an ordered series of steps that are specified in the constitution of the sovereignty. For the U.S. Congress, these steps are specified in Article 1, Sections 5 and 7 of the Constitution. Article 7 delineates the broad outlines of this process. Article 5, by giving the House of Representatives and Senate authority to "determine the rules of its proceedings," mandates the development of a set of procedures that would result in the Congress's functioning as indicated in Article 7. For a particular state or municipal legislature, at least the broad outlines of these steps would be suggested in the constitution of that state or municipality.

The steps (or decision points) that a bill must survive before becoming a statute are ordered. This ordering for a typical bill proposed in the U.S. Congress is indicated in Figure 2.5. A detailed description of the process by which legislatures create laws is being presented here because an intuitive understanding of this process is a prerequisite for influencing it. Speech-language pathologists and audiologists should obviously be interested in influencing legislation that affects both their professional functioning (e.g., licensure and third-party payments for their services under federal insurance programs) and the providing of services to the communicatively handicapped.

This graphic shows the most typical way in which proposed legislation is enacted into law. There are more complicated, as well as simpler, routes, and most bills fall by the wayside and never become law. The process is illustrated with two hypothetical bills, House bill No. 1 (HR 1) and Senate bill No. 2 (S 2). Each bill must be passed by both houses of Congress in identical form before it can become law. The path of HR 1 is traced by a solid line, that of S 2 by a broken line. However, in practice most legislation begins as similar proposals in both houses.

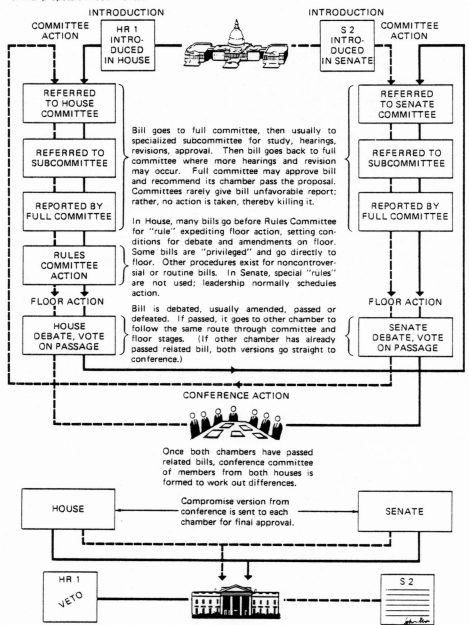

INTRODUCTION

COMMITTEE ACTION

HR 1 INTRODUCED IN HOUSE

INTRODUCTION

S 2 INTRODUCED IN SENATE

COMMITTEE ACTION

REFERRED TO HOUSE COMMITTEE

REFERRED TO SUBCOMMITTEE

REPORTED BY FULL COMMITTEE

RULES COMMITTEE ACTION

FLOOR ACTION

HOUSE DEBATE, VOTE ON PASSAGE

REFERRED TO SENATE COMMITTEE

REFERRED TO SUBCOMMITTEE

REPORTED BY FULL COMMITTEE

FLOOR ACTION

SENATE DEBATE, VOTE ON PASSAGE

Bill goes to full committee, then usually to specialized subcommittee for study, hearings, revisions, approval. Then bill goes back to full committee where more hearings and revision may occur. Full committee may approve bill and recommend its chamber pass the proposal. Committees rarely give bill unfavorable report; rather, no action is taken, thereby killing it.

In House, many bills go before Rules Committee for "rule" expediting floor action, setting conditions for debate and amendments on floor. Some bills are "privileged" and go directly to floor. Other procedures exist for noncontroversial or routine bills. In Senate, special "rules" are not used; leadership normally schedules action.

Bill is debated, usually amended, passed or defeated. If passed, it goes to other chamber to follow the same route through committee and floor stages. (If other chamber has already passed related bill, both versions go straight to conference.)

CONFERENCE ACTION

Once both chambers have passed related bills, conference committee of members from both houses is formed to work out differences.

HOUSE

Compromise version from conference is sent to each chamber for final approval.

SENATE

HR 1 VETO

S 2

Compromise version approved by both houses is sent to President who can either sign it into law or veto it and return it to Congress. Congress may override veto by a two-thirds majority vote in both houses; bill then becomes law without President's signature.

FIGURE 2.5 How a bill becomes law. (adapted from GUIDE TO CONGRESS, Second Edition. Washington, D.C.: Congressional Quarterly, Inc., 1976.)

Administrative Agencies

Administrative agencies are rule-making (lawmaking) organizations that exist in all federal, state, and municipal governments. They may be referred to as commissions, services, boards, authorities, bureaus, offices, departments, corporations, administrations, divisions, or agencies. Those in the federal government that make rules which influence the activities of speech-language pathologists and audiologists include the following:

Equal Employment Opportunity Commission
Internal Revenue Service
Occupational Safety and Health Review Commission
Department of Education (Special Education Programs)
Office of Human Development Services
Social Security Administration
Department of Veteran's Affairs

Information about these and other federal administrative agencies (including names and telephone numbers of key personnel) can be found in the *United States Government Manual,* which is published annually by the U.S. Government Printing Office.

Administrative agencies are created by the legislative and executive branches of government to develop, administer, and enforce programs they have mandated in specific areas (e.g., education of the handicapped). A state legislature, for example, might pass a bill that would regulate the activities of speech-language pathologists and audiologists by licensure. To implement it the legislature would have included in the bill provisions either for establishing a special licensure board for regulating speech, language, and hearing services or for assigning responsibility for implementation to an existing board (e.g., one responsible for administering similar laws for health-related professions). In the State of Wisconsin, for example, this responsibility was assigned to the existing board established for licensing hearing-aid dealers. Licensure boards are administrative agencies. They are responsible for the nitty-gritty of (1) developing the guidelines, or rules, that are necessary for implementing a licensure law [legislative function]; (2) evaluating the qualifications of persons who wish to be licensed under it and, if their qualifications are adequate, granting them licenses [executive function]; and (3) policing persons who have been licensed and if necessary conducting hearings that could result in suspension or revocation of their licenses [judicial function]. Almost all administrative agencies perform legislative, executive, and judicial functions (see the comments in square brackets in the preceding sentence). Thus, they do not appear to adhere to the concept of separation of powers that, judging by the Constitution, is a fundamental aspect of our form of government. (This aspect of their functioning has been challenged on constitutional grounds, but apparently not successfully.)

Administrative agencies are not mentioned directly in the Constitution. They owe their existence to the legislative and executive branches of government. Congress, theoretically, can terminate any federal administrative agency by merely passing a statute. Administrative agencies were originally established to implement legislation at relatively low cost with as few mistakes as possible. It was believed that it would be more costly to have members of Congress develop the rules for implementing a statute than to have a group of bureaucrats do it. Moreover, a group of bureaucrats with expertise in the specific subject matter area of the legislation would probably be less likely to make errors as they established rules than would members of Congress, most of whom probably would lack expertise in the subject matter. Of course, concluding that administrative agencies, because of their expertise, would be less likely to make errors in rule making than would the Congress is not the same as concluding that they would not make errors. No decision-making process can be completely error-free. Rules that are either unreasonable or undesirable (or both) have been promulgated by administrative agencies. However, rules that are viewed to be such can be challenged in the courts.

The procedure that an administrative agency follows for rule making is supposed to allow for input from any interested party. Those that federal administrative agencies are required to follow, which are summarized here, illustrate how such input can influence this process.

> The basic procedural ideas are quite simple: An agency prepares a proposed rule after whatever study and investigation and consultation it finds desirable, publishes it, invites written comments on it, reworks it in the light of the comments, and then issues the final rule. Sometimes the agency hears oral arguments. Sometimes it issues a second proposed rule. Sometimes, when issues of specific fact call for such procedures, the agency conducts a trial-type hearing on those issues. The procedure is flexible and the variations depend upon circumstances and special needs.
>
> Much experience shows that the procedure is efficient, fair, democratic, and easy. A small party may write a letter to point out how a proposed

rule will affect him, to request a slight alteration, and to make an argument. A big company may make an elaborate study, present detailed results, and ask for opportunity for its lawyers to present oral argument. The agency will summarize the main new facts and ideas and explain the reasons for the choices it makes. Anyone has the opportunity to propose changes not only in proposed rules but even in rules that have been adopted (Davis, 1977, p. 241).

The procedure that would be used by state and municipal administrative agencies for obtaining public input on proposed rules would be quite similar in most instances.

How can one keep informed about new rules being proposed by administrative agencies? For federal administrative agencies, most of these are published in a periodical distributed by the U.S. Government Printing Office known as the *Federal Register*. It also includes information about new rules that have been adopted by these agencies. Although it is almost always possible to obtain information about new rules being proposed by state and municipal administrative agencies, this information often cannot be obtained as conveniently as it can for federal ones because they are not published in a widely circulated periodical comparable to the *Federal Register*.

Rules, guidelines, and other records generated by federal agencies that are not published in the *Federal Register* can often be obtained directly from these agencies by requesting the information under the terms of the *Freedom of Information Act*. The word "often" was used because (1) this act requires the person requesting a document to specifically identify it and (2) the act contains a list of exemptions; if the agency can argue convincingly that the information being requested is covered by one or more of these exemptions, it can refuse to release it.

Why might a speech-language pathologist or audiologist request information from a federal agency under the *Freedom of Information Act?* One reason could be to obtain the full set of reviewers' comments on a grant application that he or she had submitted which was rejected if the agency refused to provide it.

Professional Organizations

Professional organizations, such as the American Speech-Language-Hearing Association, are not usually regarded as possible sources of law because they are not a component of municipal, state, or federal government. Yet they often function in this role, particularly if they certify the professional competence of their members and develop, administer, and enforce a code of ethics. The influence they exert over their members when functioning in this capacity is comparable to that exerted by an *administrative agency* over its constituents. One type of administrative agency that an organization functioning in this way is comparable to is a state occupational licensing board. In awarding its Certificates of Clinical Competence in Speech-Language Pathology and Audiology, the American Speech-Language-Hearing Association behaves similarly to such a board. It performs legislative, executive, and judicial functions: It establishes the requirements for the certificates [legislative function]; it evaluates the qualifications of persons who apply for one or both of them [executive function]; and it monitors the activities of persons who have been awarded them [judicial function].

Information about new rules under consideration by a professional organization and recently adopted rules are usually published in one of the organization's journals or newsletters. The American Speech-Language-Hearing Association publishes such information in the journal *Asha.*

HOW ARE THE LAWS THAT MAKE UP OUR LEGAL SYSTEM CATEGORIZED?

Having examined the sources from which we get the laws that make up on legal system, we shall now consider the laws themselves and specifically, some of the terms used for categorizing them. An intuitive understanding of the meanings of such terms (categories), of course, can help us understand the intended function of laws within the categories.

All rules (laws) that are intended to influence our behavior, regardless of their origin, can be assigned to one of *three* content categories: criminal, administrative, or civil (see Figure 2.6). *Criminal laws* deal with crimes, or acts against society. Such acts can be against a municipal or state government, the federal government, or the international community (e.g., genocide). Some deviations from society's behavioral expectations, or crimes, are viewed as more serious than are others. Relatively minor ones, such as parking your car in a no-parking zone, are classified as *misdemeanors;* more serious ones are classified as *felonies.* Misdemeanors usually are punishable by relatively low fines and/or relatively short terms of imprisonment. Felonies are punishable by relatively large fines, relatively long terms of imprisonment, and in some states in some extremely serious cases (such as murder), death. One is accused of committing a crime by a representative of the governmental unit against which it was supposedly committed, such as a district attorney. When a criminal case is tried by a court, it ordinarily is titled *people* versus the name of the defendant (e.g., *People v. Silverman*). This convention highlights the fact what the person is accused of doing is contrary to the interests of society—that is, the people. In such court proceedings the defendant is presumed to be innocent: He or she can be found guilty only if the people can establish guilt *beyond a shadow of a doubt.*

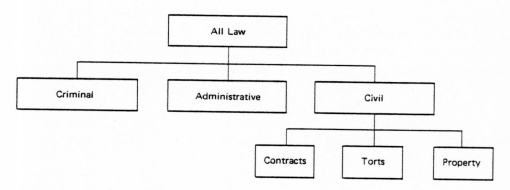

FIGURE 2.6 Some types of laws that are professionally relevant.

Administrative law deals with regulations promulgated by municipal, state, and federal administrative agencies. Information about such agencies as a source of law is presented in the preceding section of this chapter.

Civil law is concerned with the relationships between private individuals (rather than between private individuals and society, which is the concern of criminal law). We all enter into many such relationships, and when doing so we implicitly or explicitly accept restrictions and obligations. Civil law deals with those restrictions and obligations intended to protect the rights of private individuals. It makes them explicit and offers *procedures* for resolving controversies involving them. These procedures include the *civil suit,* in which "the court attempts to remedy the controversy between individuals by determining their legal rights, awarding money damages to the injured party, or directing one party to do or refrain from doing a specific act" (Grilliot, 1979, p. 23).

There are several types (categories) of civil law. Those that are professionally relevant to speech-language pathologists and audiologists include contracts, torts, and property.

Contract law is intended to facilitate interpersonal relationships. For a society to exist in which individuals are not completely self-sufficient (which would be any society) its members have to *cooperate*. Few individuals can provide for themselves more than a small number of the goods and services they require for their survival. They must rely on others for most of them. The agreement by which these goods and services are provided is known as a contract. A contract is "a promise, or set of promises, for *breach* of which the law gives a *remedy*, or the performance of which the law in some way recognizes as a *duty*" (Gifis, 1991, p. 97). The role of contracts in clinical practice is dealt with in Chapter 5.

Torts are injuries or wrongs to individuals resulting from the dangerous or unreasonable conduct of others, *that do not arise from breaching (not fulfilling) a contract,* for which courts will provide a remedy by awarding compensation. The assumption here, of course, is that the injuries or wrongs can be proven to have resulted from dangerous or unreasonable conduct by the defendant. Torts differ from crimes in that crimes are injuries or wrongs to *society*, and torts are injuries or wrongs to *private individuals.* Thus, the plaintiff (accuser) in a court case involving a crime is society—the people—and that in a court case involving a tort is a private individual. A given act, incidentally, can be viewed as both a tort and a crime if it can be proven to have caused injury to both society and a private individual (or group of individuals). The types of wrongs or injuries that one person can do to another through dangerous or unreasonable conduct (which are the types of torts) include negligence (a professionally relevant aspect of which is *malpractice*), invasion of privacy, defamation (as in saying or writing something false about another professional that results in injury to his or her reputation), infliction of mental distress, assault, battery, and trespass. Those of particular concern to clinicians are dealt with in Chapter 6.

Property law is concerned with rights of ownership. Though property law is relevant to everyone since we all own something, several aspects of it are particularly relevant to clinicians. These, which include patents, copyrights, and clinic records, are dealt with in Chapters 7 and 8.

In addition to being assignable to content categories, laws also are assignable to *function categories*. There are two such categories: substantive and procedural. *Substantive laws* are those that create, define, and regulate duties or rights and by so doing place restrictions and obligations on our behavior. Such laws tell us what we should and should not do. Almost all regulations promulgated by administrative agencies can be classified as substantive since they specify what should and should not be done to the members of a particular subpopulation, such as communicatively handicapped children. Almost all laws (statutes) created by legislatures can be classified by substantive.

Procedural laws specify how substantive laws are to be enforced. They provide the necessary machinery for enforcing duties and protecting rights prescribed by substantive laws. They specify the ground rules that the judicial branch of a government must follow to enforce the duties and protect the rights mandated by its substantive laws. An example of a procedural law is the federal *due process guaranty*. This guaranty, which is included in the Fifth Amendment, states that no person shall "be deprived of life, liberty, or property without due process of law." To deprive someone of life, liberty, or property, the federal government must *strictly* adhere to, or follow, procedures acceptable to the federal judiciary.

HOW ARE THE LAWS THAT MAKE UP OUR LEGAL SYSTEM ENFORCED?

Once a law has been created by action of a legislature, an administrative agency, a court decision, or a rule-making body of a professional organization (e.g., the Legislative Council of the American Speech-Language-Hearing Association), it is necessary to provide a mechanism through which it can be enforced. Without such a mechanism, the law is unlikely to have its intended impact on behavior. People tend to be unwilling to obey laws restricting their activities if they do not *anticipate* adverse consequences to themselves for not obeying them. In fact, if the probability of a particular law's being obeyed is to be maximized, the persons to whom it applies must *expect* the negative consequences of not obeying it to outweigh the potential benefits of doing so. The words *anticipate* and *expect* are italicized to highlight the role of anticipation of negative consequences in the enforcement of laws. If, for example, we feel that failure to obey a law could result in damage to our reputation, we are likely to obey that law. Also, fear of the consequences of a tax audit can influence how a person completes an income tax form.

On municipal, state, and federal levels, the *courts* are the principal institutions that enforce laws. They not only enforce statutes enacted by legislatures, but law created by judges (common law) and regulations promulgated by administrative agencies. Some federal administrative agencies, such as the Internal Revenue Service, have their own courts which interface with the U.S. Court of Appeals (see Figure 2.4).

The mechanism by which a *belief* that a law has been broken is brought to the attention of a court is known as a *lawsuit*, or *suit*. The person (or group) who initiates the suit is referred to as the *plaintiff*. The plaintiff in a *civil suit* usually is one person but can be a group of persons. The latter would occur in a *class-action suit* — for example, all persons in the State of Wisconsin who purchased a particular model of automobile that did not contain the engine specified in their contracts might as a group (or class) sue to force the manufacturer to give them cars containing this engine.

The plaintiff in a *criminal suit* is the *people* — that is, the population of a municipality, state, or nation. In a criminal suit in a municipal court, for example, the plaintiff would be the people who reside in that municipality.

The person or group whom the plaintiff accuses of breaking the law — the person or group being sued — is referred to as the *defendant*. The defendant in a civil suit can be either an individual or a group. Groups that can be sued include corporations, governmental units, voluntary organizations, institutions (e.g., hospitals), and groups consisting of several professionals of whom the plaintiff was a client or patient (which can occur in a malpractice suit). The defendant is a *criminal suit* while usually an individual can be a group (e.g., a corporation).

The distinction between plaintiff and defendant in a civil suit may not be sharp. This is because the defendant can initiate a *countersuit* against the plaintiff. The defendant, for example, can accuse the plaintiff of committing a tort. Thus, in the countersuit the defendant becomes the plaintiff and the plaintiff the defendant.

The plaintiff and defendant in a suit are each ordinarily represented by one or more attorneys. Occasionally, the plaintiff or defendant may choose not to be represented by an attorney. A person acting as his or her own attorney is referred to as a *pro se litigant*. (*Litigant* is a legal term for an active party, or participant, in a lawsuit — a plaintiff or defendant.) The only type of lawsuit in which the parties customarily function as *pro se litigants* is that heard by a *small claims court.* Unless a litigant in any other type of lawsuit has had considerable legal training, he or she will probably decrease the probability of achieving the desired outcome as a plaintiff and/or defendant by acting as his or her own attorney.

A defendant in a lawsuit is almost always charged an *hourly fee* by his or her attorney. The fee is determined, at least in part, by the amount of time the attorney spends on the suit. The attorney would expect to be paid regardless of whether the wins or loses the suit. Occasionally, an attorney may represent a defendant without compensation to advance a social cause (i.e., for the public good): He or she is said to be representing the party *pro bono publico.*

The fee the attorney charges the *plaintiff* in a lawsuit may be hourly, or it may be based on the size of the award the plaintiff receives if he or she wins the suit (Ostberg, 1990). When the latter arrangement is used, the attorney receives a percentage (perhaps a third) of the money the client is awarded. If he or she loses the suit, the attorney receives no money. Obviously, attorneys are unlikely to accept such an arrangement unless they believe that their clients have a good chance of winning a substantial award.

Judicial Remedies

Those initiating a civil suit do so for the purpose of forcing someone to do something. They seek a *remedy* to a conflict they are having with someone—a conflict they have been unable to resolve to their satisfaction. People usually do not initiate suits to resolve conflicts until they have exhausted other possibilities. Because of the cost in time, money, and "stress," having a dispute settled by a court should be viewed as a last resort.

When a plaintiff initiates a suit, he or she must specify the remedy being sought—that is, what he or she wants the court to order the defendant to do. A court can order several types of remedies in civil suits. These are summarized in Figure 2.7 and discussed in the following paragraphs.

There are two main types of *judicial remedies:* equity and common law. The first, *equity,* is concerned primarily with *injunctions.* These either mandate a defendant to carry out some specific activity or prohibit a defendant from doing something. An example of a *mandatory injunction* would be a court order to a school district to pay the tuition of a deaf child to attend a private school when the district had no classes for such a

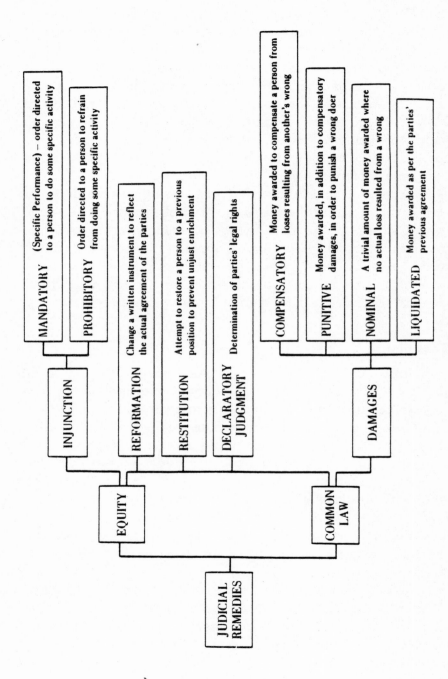

FIGURE 2.7 Actions that a court can take on behalf of the plaintiff in a civil suit. (From Harold J. Grilliot, INTRODUCTION TO LAW AND THE LEGAL SYSTEM, Second Edition. Copyright 1979 by Houghton Mifflin Company. Reprinted by permission of the publisher.)

child. In this suit the parents probably would have been the plaintiff and the school district the defendant. If the school district had been paying the child's tuition and planned to stop, the parents might have sought a *prohibitory injunction*, which would be a court order prohibiting the district from discontinuing payment of the child's tuition.

The second type of remedy, *common law*, is concerned primarily with the awarding of *damages* (see Figure 2.7). Here the plaintiff seeks money from the defendant in compensation for an "injury" (or "injuries") that the plaintiff feels was done to him or her by the defendant. The plaintiff can seek several types of damages. The first would be *compensatory damages*. Such damages are intended to compensate the plaintiff for the injury received from the defendant. At least some of the damages a plaintiff would seek in a *malpractice suit* would be of this type. The rationale underlying the awarding of compensatory damages is that the action of the defendant resulted in the plaintiff's sustaining a loss, and he or she should be awarded damages of a magnitude that would compensate for this loss.

Punitive damages, the second type of damages, are awarded to the plaintiff *in addition to* compensatory damages to punish the defendant. A court may award punitive damages to a plaintiff when

> the wrong done to him was aggravated by circumstances of violence, oppression, malice, fraud, or wanton or wicked conduct on the part of the defendant, and are intended to solace the plaintiff for mental anguish, laceration of his feelings, shame, degradation, or other aggravations of the original wrong, or else to punish the defendant for his evil behavior or to make an example of him (Black, 1968, pp. 467–468).

A court ordinarily will not award punitive damages without strong evidence that such damages are warranted.

The third type of damages, *nominal damages*, are small amounts of money awarded to plaintiffs when the wrong done to them did not result in an actual injury, although technically their rights were invaded. A court makes such an award to a plaintiff to acknowledge the wrong. Suppose, for example, an audiologist agrees to buy a customized audiometer for $10,000. When the audiometer is delivered, he refuses to accept it—in other words, he breaches the contract. The manufacturer sells the audiometer to another audiologist for $10,000 and sues the one who originally ordered it for *breach of contract*. While the audiologist is technically guilty of breach of contract, the manufacturer did not sustain any significant financial loss because the audiometer was sold for the same amount of money. Thus, the only damages that a court would be likely to award would be nominal ones. Some persons who have been technically wronged will not initiate a lawsuit, in least in part, because the amount of money they are likely to be awarded will be offset by the fees they will be charged by their attorneys.

A fourth type of damages, *liquidated damages*, is a certain amount of money specified in a contract that the party who breaches the contract agrees to pay to the other party in the contract. A contract with a construction company for building a communicative disorders treatment center may include a clause that states that the building is to be ready for occupancy by a certain date and that if it is not, the company will have to pay a penalty. Such a clause would be included to motivate the contractor to live up to his, her, or its (if a corporation) contractual obligations.

In addition to issuing injunctions and awarding damages, courts offer several other types of remedies (see Figure 2.7). These include reformation, restitution, and declaratory judgment. *Reformation* (revision) can be ordered by a court when a written contract does not accurately reflect the agreement between the parties because of error, fraud, or ambiguous language. The assumption is that it would be unconscionable to force persons to abode by the terms of a written contract, when the document was not an *accurate map of the territory* it was supposed to represent — that is, the actual agreement between the parties (Korzybski, 1933). One strategy that can be used for motivating someone who had you sign a contract that you later discovered did not accurately "map" your agreement to modify it is to threaten to seek reformation from a court unless he or she voluntarily agrees to do so.

Restitution can be ordered by a court if a plaintiff has been unjustly deprived of a right or property. It is intended to prevent the unjust enrichment of the person who deprived him or her of the property or right. Restitution may or may not involve money. It can include any tangible or intangible property. Restitution involving money differs from damages in that restitution focuses on the *defendant's unjust gain* and damages on the *plaintiff's unjust loss.*

A person who seeks a *declaratory judgment* seeks clarification from a court about what the law is in a particular situation or about the meaning of the law in that situation. A person may also seek a judgment from a court regarding the *constitutionality* of a statute passed by a legislature. If a legislature passed a statute that made an activity a person engaged in illegal, the person might seek a declaratory judgment, thereby asking a court to declare the statute unconstitutional and hence unenforceable. If, for example, a child's parents felt that he or she was entitled to but was denied funding for a communication prosthesis from a particular state or federal insurance program, they might seek a declaratory judgment from a court to clarify the situation. The *threat* of doing so may motivate an agency to find a "face-saving" way to provide the person with what he or she is requesting. The reason is that if the court makes a declaratory judgment, it may not only have to provide the person requesting it with what is being asked for (e.g., a communication prosthesis), but others who are in similar circumstances as well.

Steps in a Civil Lawsuit

If a speech-language pathologist or audiologist wanted to seek one of the judicial remedies discussed in the previous section, what steps would he or she have to take? The components of a typical civil lawsuit are summarized in Figure 2.8 and described in the paragraphs that follow.

The process that initiates a civil lawsuit begins with the occurrence of an *action* for which there is a judicial remedy. Such actions would include failure to live up to the terms of a contract, reproducing copy-righted material (e.g., computer software) without permission of the copyright owner, releasing information in a person's clinic folder with-out the person's permission, and denying a person services to which he or she is entitled by law.

A person may become aware that he or she has been legally wronged immediately after the action or some time thereafter. Time may elapse because the person is unaware that a judicial remedy is available to rectify the wrong done to him or her. (One of the objectives of this book is heighten your awareness of the judicial remedies that are available to you.) Unfortunately, if too much time elapses between when a person is wronged and when he or she becomes aware of the possibility of a legal remedy, he or she may be unable to initiate a suit because of the *statute of limitations.* A person does not have an unlimited amount of time in which to *initiate* a suit. He or she must do it within a certain number of years. The amount of time allowed depends on the nature of the wrong. For example, a person usually has a shorter period of time to initiate a suit for a tort than for failure to live up to the obligations imposed by a contract (Fisher, 1977). The main objective of the statute of limitations is

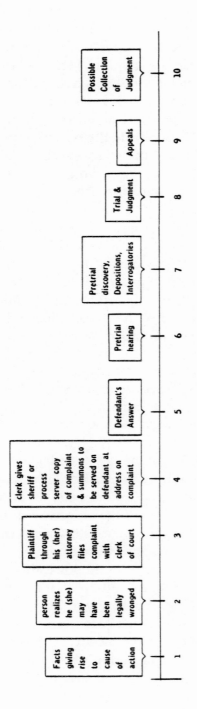

FIGURE 2.8 Steps in a civil lawsuit. (Reproduced with permission from INTRODUCTION TO THE LEGAL SYSTEM, Second Edition by Bruce D. Fisher. Copyright 1977 by West Publishing Company. All rights reserved.)

the maintenance of *community peace.* The sooner conflicts are settled, the sooner people can resume their usual activities. Also, if people were allowed to initiate suits long after they were wronged, the courts might be unable to obtain some information they needed because evidence was lost and witnesses moved away or died.

The party to the lawsuit who will raise the issue of the statute of limitations is the defendant. If the defendant can convince the court that the plaintiff has waited too long to initiate the suit, he or she can avoid having to be a party to it. The attorney for the defendant may raise the issue of the statute of limitations at the beginning of the lawsuit in an effort to end the suit.

Once a person has become aware of having been legally wronged and decides to seek a judicial remedy—to initiate a lawsuit—he or she will discuss it with an attorney. (For a discussion of factors to consider when shopping for an attorney see Ostberg, 1990.) This, of course, assumes that the person decided not to act *pro se* (i.e., as his or her own attorney). If the attorney feels after hearing the complaint and possibly doing some informal investigation the suit being proposed has merit and the person is likely to be awarded the remedy being sought, he or she is likely to agree to represent the person on either a flat fee, hourly fee, or contingency fee basis (see Ostberg, 1990 for a discussion of advantages and disadvantages of these fee arrangements). The attorney will tend draft a *written complaint* that indicates why the client (the plaintiff in the suit being initiated) believes he or she was legally wronged by the defendant, and what judicial remedy is being sought. The original and two copies are delivered to the *clerk of the court* in which the plaintiff intends to initiate the suit. The clerk stamps the three copies with the date and time of day, keeps the original, returns one copy to the plaintiff, and gives the third copy to an *official process server* along with a *summons,* which directs the defendant to appear in court to answer the complaint. The process server delivers the copy of the complaint and the summons to the person (or organization) who will be the defendant in the suit. This serves as official notification to the defendant that he or she is being sued.

Once the defendant recovers somewhat from the shock of being sued, he or she will hire an attorney (assuming that the person does not choose to be a *pro se* litigant). The attorney will draft a *written answer* to the plaintiff's complaint and will file it with the clerk of the court in which the plaintiff initiated the suit. The defendant ordinarily is given a relatively short period of time to file an answer, usually thirty days. (The date-time-of-day stamp that was placed on the complaint by the clerk of the court lets the defendant know when the deadline for filing is.) The defendant's version of the incident giving rise to the suit is indicated in the answer. Also may be indicated a summary of *procedural reasons* why the defendant feels the plaintiff should not be awarded the remedy he or she is seeking (such as the plaintiff waiting too long to initiate a suit because of the statute of limitations). If the defendant fails to file an answer by the deadline without having an extraordinarily good excuse, the plaintiff wins the suit.

In the period between when the defendant files his or her answer and the beginning of the trial, both the plaintiff and defendant gather evidence to support their contentions. Much of this evidence will be documented by the statements of persons who have knowledge that supports one or more of them. The statements can be made under oath at the trial and/or under oath prior to the trial during a face-to-face questioning session. Statements of the latter type are referred to as *depositions.* They can be solicited by either the attorney for the plaintiff or the attorney for the defendant. An attorney may choose to document the evidence in a witness's statement by a pre-trial deposition for any of several reasons — for example, the witness will be unavailable for the trial or the attorney wants to statement of the relevant information while it is still fresh in the witness's mind. The period between a suit being initiated and the trial can be two or more years (Charles & Kennedy, 1985). Attorneys for both parties are usually present while a deposition is being taken. Statements made while a deposition is being taken are recorded and transcribed, usually by a court reporter.

Another strategy that plaintiffs and defendants use for gathering evidence to support their contentions is requesting answers to *interrogatories.* Interrogatories are written questions that are submitted by one party to the other. The party to whom they are submitted usually is given thirty days to answer them (Feuer, 1990). The defendant's attorney, for example, may ask the plaintiff's to identify the specific allegations claimed in the complaint and/or to indicate if they plan to use an expert witness and if they do, what his or her testimony is expected to state. And the plaintiff's interrogatories may ask the defendant to describe the treatment given (if it is a malpractice suit) and/or if he or she plans to use expert witnesses what they will testify.

There are several other strategies, or *discovery devices,* that attorneys for plaintiffs and defendants may use for gathering data to support their contentions. One is a request for the production of documents relevant to the case (e.g., evaluation and progress reports). The requesting party submits a list of items for production to the other side. The receiving party may object and refuse to produce a document because he or she claims it is not relevant. Such objections are ultimately decided by the judge.

A second such device that may be used by a defendant in a case in which the plaintiff claims that he or she was physically or psychologically harmed by the defendant (e.g., in a malpractice case), is to have the plaintiff examined by an independent appropriate health-care professional. This examination is usually performed to refute the plaintiff's testimony about the extent of injuries. If, for example, the claimed injury was to hearing, an appropriate independent professional to perform the examination would be a *forensic audiologist* (Kramer & Armbruster, 1982).

Prior to the trial each party to the lawsuit usually has an opportunity to find out, or *discover*, the sorts of evidence the other party has and is likely to use. Also prior to the trial the attorneys for the plaintiff and defendant may have a conference with the judge who will be presiding at the trial. Such a conference can reduce trial time because it can pinpoint what each side would have to prove in order to win the suit. Also, information obtained during the conference and discovery process could convince the defendant that he or she would have little or no chance of winning the suit and could, thereby, motivate the defendant to reach an *out-of-court settlement* with the plaintiff. Or it could convince the plaintiff that he or she would have little or no chance of being awarded the remedy being sought from the court and could, thereby, motivate the plaintiff to drop the suit. Out-of-court settlements are desirable because they save both parties to a suit the expense and emotional strain of a trial. They also are desirable from the court's point of view. Most courts are overloaded with cases, and as a consequence a relatively long period of time often elapses between the initiation of a suit and the trial. The higher the percentage of cases assigned to a court that can be settled without a trial, the shorter this time period.

If the plaintiff and defendant are unable to settle their dispute before their suit is scheduled to be tried, they will become participants in a complex competitive team game known as a *trial*. The arena is a courtroom. The main participants, beside the plaintiff and defendant, will be their attorneys, their witnesses, the judge, and the jury. The plaintiff and defendant may agree to play the game without a jury, in which case the judge assumes the jury's functions.

There are two teams. One consists of the plaintiff, his or her attorney (or attorneys), and witnesses. The other consists of the defendant, his or her attorney (or attorneys), and witnesses.

The *judge* ultimately decides which team wins the game; and if it is the plaintiff's team, what the prize—the judicial remedy—should be. The judge also functions as *referee* and sees to it that both teams obey the rules of the game. The judge settles disputes when one team charges the other with violating a rule (or rules) and as referee enforces the rules of the game in an appropriate and evenhanded manner. If the judge fails to enforce the rules in such a manner and the decision is appealed to a higher, or *appellate* court, it can be reversed on this basis. Obviously, the team that lost the game would be the one that would attempt to demonstrate that the rules were not enforced in an appropriate and evenhanded manner. The team that won would be unlikely to question the enforcement of the rules, even if they felt that the manner in which the judge did it was blatantly inappropriate and unevenhanded.

A judge, like other human beings, can make mistakes and be biased. A person becomes a judge either by being appointed or elected. If the means was appointment it could have been primarily for political reasons. If a judge was elected, it could have been primarily on the basis of the image he or she communicated to the voters. While the *office of judge* certainly should be respected, a person holding that office should not be regarded as superhuman.

The *jury* in a civil case assists the judge in deciding questions of fact. The plaintiff and defendant probably will present at least somewhat different versions of what happened. The function of the jury is to decide who is most likely to be telling the truth. They are supposed to weigh the evidence presented by each party to support its position on each question of fact and then to decide which position is best supported by the evidence. The jury bases its decision on what is presented. If the attorney for one party does not adequately present the evidence that supports his or her client's position, the client could lose the suit on this basis. Hence, the relative competency of the attorneys representing the parties can have a significant impact on who wins.

The verdict rendered by a jury in a civil suit does not have to be accepted by the judge, at least theoretically (Fisher, 1977). If a jury renders a verdict that appears to be completely at odds with the evidence, the party who is hurt by it can ask the court for a *judgment notwithstanding the verdict.* If the judge agrees that the verdict was not consistent with the evidence, he or she can disregard it and decide in favor of the moving party. Of course, the judge's decision is likely to be appealed by the other party.

The attorneys representing the parties to a lawsuit can be viewed as team captains and coaches. If the parties do not choose to be *pro se* litigants, each will empower one or more attorneys to present his or her case to the judge and jury—that is to speak for him or her. Litigants retain the right, however, to discharge their attorney(s) at any point in the proceedings if dissatisfied with how the case is being presented. The attorney, or attorneys, representing each party assume the major responsibility for the planning and presentation of the client's case (and thus function as the captain of the client's team). They "coach" the witnesses who will provide evidence to support their client's case. Attorneys as *officers of the court* are ethically bound when functioning in this latter role not to encourage witnesses to lie, or *perjure,* themselves. Their primary responsibility is to present the strongest case they can to support their client's position in the suit and to make certain that the manner in which the court proceedings are conducted by the judge does not violate their client's constitutional guarantees of *procedural due process.*

The witnesses an attorney can use to support a client's case are of two types. The first consists of persons having *direct knowledge* of some aspect of the action giving rise to the suit whose testimony would be expected to provide evidence that supports one or more of aspects of his or her case. Such testimony usually consists of a description of what the witness heard and/or saw. (It also may include a description of what he or she touched, smelled, or tasted.)

The second type is referred to as an *expert witness.* Those functioning in this role are usually licensed or certified as competent to engage in a profession such as medicine, clinical psychology, speech-language pathology, or audiology. Because of their training and experience in a particular discipline, they can be viewed as experts whose *opinions* on matters relevant to that discipline are likely to be accurate enough that they are admissible as evidence. A speech-language pathologist, for example, might be asked to evaluate an aphasic and to testify (give an expert opinion) about whether the person is able to communicate well enough to continue to manage his or her financial affairs. And an audiologist might be asked to evaluate a factory worker who has developed a presumably job-related, noise-induced hearing loss and to give an expert opinion about how much the worker is handicapped by it. Such testimony could assist a worker's compensation court in deciding how much to award him or her. The expert witness is dealt with further in Chapter 11.

The two types of witnesses that are described in the preceding paragraphs are asked to testify by one of the parties to the suit. Sometimes an individual or organization who is not a party to the suit and is not asked to testify by one of parties to it wishes to do so. Such a person or organization would submit an *amicus curiae (i.e., "friend of the court") brief.* This is done "to aid the court in gaining information which it needs to make a proper decision or to urge a particular result on behalf of the public or a private interest of third parties who will be indirectly affected by the resolution of the dispute" (Gifis, 1991, p. 22). ASHA, for example, filed such a brief in a suit involving a hearing aid dealer who was referring to himself as an "audiologist" (Ohio Federal District Court allows ASHA to file as *Amicus Curiae,* 1991).

Now that the roles of the participants in the game (trial) have been described, we will consider the *rules* by which the game is played. A civil trial "game" consists of a series of events, or activities, that are ordered in a particular manner. These will be summarized here. (The primary source for the information presented in this discussion was Grilliot, 1979, pp. 245–271.)

The first major event or activity in a civil trial is the selection of the *jury.* The members of a jury are selected from a pool of people (usually registered voters from the community in which the court is located) who were told to be at the courthouse and available for jury duty (Wishman, 1986).

At the beginning of the selection process, a group of prospective jurors are questioned by the attorneys for both parties and by the judge. The purpose of the questioning is to determine whether there are grounds for believing that any of them are unlikely to be *impartial* (without prejudice or bias) when rendering a verdict. The attorneys for both parties can challenge the potential impartiality of as many as they wish, and those that the judge agrees are apt to be biased or prejudiced will be replaced. Included here would be persons who are acquainted with any of the parties to the suit or any of the witnesses who will be testifying. In addition, each party is given a limited number of *peremptory challenges.* These can be used to remove prospective jurors without having to show cause. As prospective jurors are removed through successful challenges, they are replaced with others from the pool. The examination-replacement process continues until an adequate number have been selected to form a jury. The jury members are then sworn in.

The attorneys for both parties to a lawsuit seek to form a jury that at the very least could be expected to be impartial and ideally would tend to be biased in favor of their client (Wishman, 1986). Those for both sides would have in mind the profile for such a jury while engaging in the selection process. By using challenges (particularly preemptory challenges) wisely, each will attempt to form a jury the profile of which will approximate his or her ideal one as closely as possible (see Wenke, 1989). Obviously, if one party's attorney was more knowledgeable than the other's about the attributes of jurors who would be most likely to believe his or her client, the resulting jury would be more likely to be sympathetic to one side than to the other. Thus, it is possible for the winner to be determined by the first move of the game (trial).

The next major event that occurs in a civil trial is the *opening statements* of the plaintiff's and defendant's attorneys. The plaintiff's attorney in it explains the facts of the case to the judge and jury from his or her client's perspective, including an explanation of the legal theory that would warrant the court's awarding the remedy being sought. The attorney also would indicate what he or she intends to prove during the trial. If the defendant's attorney chooses to make an opening statement, it will deal with these topics from his or her client's perspective. The opening statements, therefore, "set the stage" for what is to follow.

Following completion of the opening statements, the attorney for the plaintiff presents his or her client's case. To win the suit and be awarded the remedy, the plaintiff must present evidence to prove those allegations made in the *complaint* that are disputed by the defendant. Admissible evidence would include relevant documents, "fact" testimony from witnesses, and opinion testimony from expert witnesses. If an ordinary witness (one who has documents or knowledge of facts that would support the plaintiff's case) refuses to voluntarily surrender the documents or testify, he or she can be ordered to do so by the court (judge). The court would issue an order that is referred to as a *subpoena duces tecum*. "A subpoena duces tecum is a written order commanding a person to appear, give testimony, and bring all documents, papers, books or records described in the subpoena" (Feuer, 1990, pp. 175–176). If the person to whom the subpoena is issued disregards it, he or she can be punished for *contempt of court.* The documents subpoenaed could be clinical or research records (Holder, 1989).

The defendant's attorney usually will attempt to discredit (or refute) each item of evidence presented by the plaintiff's attorney. If the defendant's attorney is successful, the plaintiff *should* lose the suit. (Unfortunately, good guys sometimes lose in courts of law.) The defendant's attorney will question the relevance and credibility of the documents the plaintiff's attorney introduces, the interpretation that is being given to them, or both. The defendant's attorney will *cross-examine* the plaintiff's "fact" witnesses in an attempt to raise questions about the credibility of their testimony in the minds of the judge and members of the jury and will also cross-examine the plaintiff's expert witnesses (if any) in an attempt to cast doubt on the credibility of their opinions. The defense attorney may even produce expert witnesses who will question the validity of the opinions of the plaintiff's expert witnesses. While perhaps unable to prove that the opinions of the defendant's experts are more credible than those of the plaintiff's, the defendant's attorney can at least suggest to the judge and jury that experts disagree and, hence, little weight should be given to the testimony of the plaintiff's expert witnesses.

After the plaintiff's presentation has been made, the defendant's attorney may ask the judge for an *involuntary dismissal* of the suit on the grounds that the plaintiff failed to prove the allegations in the complaint. If the judge agrees to grant this motion, the trial ends and the plaintiff loses. If the judge refuses to grant it, the trial continues.

The attorney for the defendant will attempt to prove the allegations he or she made in the *answer* to the defendant's complaint by presenting evidence. He or she will use the same types of evidence as did the plaintiff's attorney, including documents, "fact" witnesses, and expert witnesses. The attorney for the plaintiff will have an opportunity to cross-examine defense witnesses and challenge the credibility of documents the defense introduced as evidence.

After the defendant's presentation has been completed, the plaintiff's attorney has an opportunity to *rebut* the defendant's case. This ordinarily is his or her last opportunity to introduce new evidence.

After the rebuttal, the defendant's attorney is given an opportunity for a *rejoinder* to attempt to refute new evidence that was introduced during it. This ordinarily is the defendant's last opportunity to introduce new evidence.

At this point in the trial (or at any future point prior to the case's being submitted to the jury) either party may make a motion for a *directed verdict*. When attorneys for plaintiffs make this motion, they are indicating they feel their case is so strong that no reasonable jury could decide against them. When attorneys for defendants make this motion, they are indicating that they feel the plaintiff's case has no merit. If the judge grants the motion, the moving party will win the suit without it being submitted to the jury. Obviously, a judge would be unlikely to grant a motion for a directed verdict unless the case for granting the motion was extremely strong. The party that lost the suit probably would appeal the decision on this basis, and if the judge could not justify granting the motion, the decision would be likely to be reversed by the appellate court reviewing it. If the judge refuses to grant the motion for a directed verdict, the trial continues.

Both parties now present their *closing arguments*. This ordinarily will be their last opportunity to convince the judge and jury (particularly the latter) of what they need to in order to win. The plaintiff's attorney presents closing arguments first, but he or she may reserve some time for a rebuttal following the defendant's closing arguments. Both attorneys will summarize their cases and will indicate to the jury why they should reach the verdict desired by their clients.

Following the completion of closing arguments, the suit is ready to be presented to the jury. Before the jury begins its deliberations, the judge gives the jurors instructions. He or she summarizes the case, explains the substantive law that applies to it, and indicates what type of verdict is desired—general or special. If a *general verdict* is requested, the jury will decide who won the suit. If they decide for a plaintiff who is seeking damages, they also may make a recommendation concerning the amount of damages to be awarded. If the judge requests a *special verdict*, the jury will answer certain questions pertaining to facts on which the parties to the suit do not agree. The facts generated by the jury in its answers to these questions will be incorporated by the judge into the decision. How the judge words the questions obviously can influence the jury's answers and thereby the ultimate outcome of the case. The general verdict is preferred by many legal scholars for this reason.

After being instructed by the judge, the jury will leave the courtroom and *begin its deliberation*. It will continue its deliberation until its members are able to reach agreement on a verdict or until it becomes obvious that they will be unable to do so (i.e., that the jury will be a *hung jury*).

Once the jury has reached a verdict, the leader presents it in writing to the judge who, in turn, informs both parties to the suit.

At this point—that is, before the judge renders judgment—the attorney for the party who probably would lose the suit if the jury's verdict were adhered to may file a motion to have the verdict set aside (i.e., a motion for a *judgment notwithstanding the verdict of the jury*) or for a new trial. A judge would be unlikely to grant either motion unless there was clearly something wrong with the manner in which the jury reached its verdict. If, for example, there was evidence that one or more members of the jury had been coerced into voting in a particular way, this would be grounds for a judge to grant a request for a new trial.

If the judge refused to grant a motion for a new trial or for a judgment not withstanding the verdict of the jury or if no such motions were made, he or she would at this point in the proceedings *render judgment* by declaring in writing who won the suit and, if the winner was the plaintiff, by indicating the remedy being awarded—that is, indicating what the defendant is ordered to do or to refrain from doing. If the defendant does not voluntarily do what is ordered by the judge (e.g., pay damages), the plaintiff can seek an *order of execution* to force the defendant to do it.

The party losing the suit can appeal the judgment to an appellate court if dissatisfied with it. If the case was tried in a federal court, the appeal would be made to the U.S. Court of Appeals. If it was tried in a state court, the appeal would be made to the intermediate appellate court in that state court system. The party initiating the appeal would claim that *procedural errors* were made by the court (particularly the judge) during the trial that affected the outcome. If the judges in the appellate court agreed to review the case, they would examine a transcript of the courtroom proceedings to determine whether the proper legal rules had been applied. If they detect an error (or errors) that could have affected the outcome, they are likely to reverse the decision of the trial court and order it to retry the case, applying the correct procedures. If the appellate court affirms the trial court's decision, the party *may be able* to appeal the trial court judgment to higher appellate courts, including the U.S. Supreme Court.

The legal fees for an appellate court appeal can be high. Those losing a suit may decide against appealing the court decision even if they feel there are excellent grounds for doing so because of the expense involved.

A court judgment ordinarily is not carried out until the appeal process has been completed. A defendant losing a suit who wants to delay having to comply with the court judgment can do so by making all possible appeals. This process can take many years (possibly 10 or more). A corporation or governmental unit that loses a suit in which it was the defendant may use such a strategy. While its appeals are being made, it may attempt to convince the plaintiff to accept less money than was ordered by the court in return for ending the appeal process and paying him or her immediately (this would be a type of out-of-court settlement).

Perhaps one of the best ways to develop an intuitive understanding of what occurs during a civil trial is to observe several. Most trial judges will permit interested members of the public to observe in their courtrooms. Another way to develop such an understanding is to read detailed, dramatic narratives of such trials. An excellent one is in the book *Defendant* (Charles & Kennedy, 1985) which details a medical malpractice trial.

The Administrative Hearing

Speech-language pathologists and audiologists (particularly the former) probably are more likely to become involved in administrative hearings than in civil suits. They may, for example, be asked to testify as ordinary or expert witnesses at a hearing instigated by the parents of a child who has a communicative disorder in which they are seeking to force the school system to modify the child's program in a way that they feel would more adequately meet his or her special educational needs. Such hearings (referred to as *due process hearings*) have been held to enforce provisions of P.L. 94-142 (Downey, 1980a, 1980b), which mandated school systems to provide "a free, appropriate public education in the least restrictive environment" for all children for whom they are responsible. (For further information about this law, see Appendix C.)

Administrative hearings are conducted under the auspices of an administrative agency. With respect to the due process hearings that are a component of the enforcement mechanism for P.L. 94-142, the administrative agency under whose auspices such hearings are conducted is the local public school board (or local administrative agency of which it is a part).

An administrative hearing can be a means to an end or an end in itself. It can be a means for resolving issues in dispute or it can be a step in the process that terminates with the initiation of a civil suit. Most are resolved at the administrative hearing level.

An administrative hearing tends to be a *more economical* procedure for settling a dispute than a court trial for several reasons. First, a *hearing officer* rather than a judge presides. A hearing officer typically is neither a judge nor an attorney. He or she is supposed to be a *neutral person* (i.e., one who is not an employee of the agency under whose auspices the hearing is being held and has no personal or professional interests— "agendas"—that could conflict with his or her being objective) who has expertise on the issues under dispute and knows how to conduct a hearing. (The person probably would have learned how to conduct a hearing by attending a workshop for prospective hearing officers sponsored by the agency under whose auspices he or she would conduct them if requested.) Responsibilities of a hearing officer can be summarized as follows:

> A hearing officer at an administrative hearing is charged with the duty of insuring that: the hearing is conducted in an orderly and concise fashion, parties are able to present witnesses who have relevant testimony, relevant evidence is introduced into the record, and rulings are made on objections posed by the parties during the course of the hearing. The hearing officer assumes these duties in order to assure that the parties are afforded procedural due process and to assure that a clear and concise record (transcripts plus exhibits) of the hearing is created. A transcript which is clear and intelligible is essential because such a transcript serves as an aid to the hearing officer in the writing of his [or her] report and, should appeal be taken . . . serves as a basis for the . . . ruling on the merits of the appeal. (Reprinted from an unpublished document that has been used by the Wisconsin Department of Public Instruction for training hearing officers.)

A second reason why an administrative hearing tends to be more economical than a trial is that a jury is not used. A hearing officer assumes the responsibilities of both judge and jury in a civil trial.

A third reason why an administrative hearing tends to be more economical than a trial is that the arena in which it is conducted is an ordinary conference room. Also the hearing officer (partially because of where hearings are conducted) swears in witnesses and performs other functions that are performed by court personnel (e.g., the *bailiff*) during a trial.

An administrative hearing is a legal forum conducted by rules quite similar to those used for conducting a civil trial. All testimony is given under oath. Both parties have the right to cross-examine each other's witnesses and to attempt to refute each other's documentary evidence.

Both parties have the right to be represented by an attorney. Both parties have the right to subpoena documentary evidence and the testimony of reluctant witnesses. And the entire proceedings usually are recorded, either with an audiotape recorder or by a court stenographer.

The structure of an administrative hearing tends to be quite similar to that of a civil trial. Both parties begin by presenting opening statements in which they summarize the allegations they will attempt to prove. Following this, each party presents its case—that is, the evidence supporting its allegations, which could include documents and the testimony of ordinary and expert witnesses. The parties are then given an opportunity to present rebuttal evidence following which they make their closing statements.

When closing the hearing the hearing officer usually specifies the date by which he or she will present a copy of the *written decision* to the parties. The party against whom he or she decides can appeal the decision. In some instances the first level of appeal will be within the agency under whose auspices the hearing was conducted; in others it will be in the courts. (For further information about the structure of administrative hearings, see Downey, 1980a, 1980b.)

Chapter III

PROFESSIONAL ETHICS AND LAW

There is no sharp boundary between law and ethics—the two are not mutually exclusive. Our views about ethics and morality both influence the content of the laws that make up our legal system and the likelihood of these laws being obeyed. Also, an ethical code—such as that of the American Speech-Language-Hearing Association—contains prohibitions that are intended to prevent practitioners from committing *torts*, such as slander (see Chapter 6). My overall objective in this chapter is to increase your awareness of ethical considerations in clinical practice.

RELATIONSHIP BETWEEN ETHICS AND LAW

Ethics (or morality) influences law, which in turn influences how we perceive behavior from an ethical perspective (see Figure 3.1). Hence, ethics is not an entity that is separate from law but one of the forces that has and will continue to shape laws at all levels in our legal system.

Individuals in our society (as in all others) are encouraged to behave ethically (morally) in their interactions with others. We usually try to avoid interacting with persons who we feel are not behaving in this manner. This is particularly true for persons from whom we purchase goods and services.

What do we mean when we say that someone's behavior is unethical or immoral? First, we may mean that some aspects of the person's behavior do not conform to our internal standard for what constitutes moral or ethical behavior. Here we are not *describing* behavior. We are making *value judgments* about it. We are saying that it is not what we regard as fair, right, or good (see the discussion of *natural law* in Chapter 2). Unfortunately, not everyone agrees on what is fair, right, or good. Thus, the same act can be viewed as ethical by one person and as unethical by another. Also, a person's internal standard for what is fair, right, or good may not remain constant over time. A person may view a given act as ethical at one point in time and as unethical at another. Furthermore,

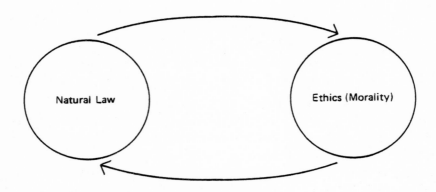

FIGURE 3.1 relationship between ethics and law.

a person's internal standard for what is fair, right, or good may vary on a *situational basis*. Thus, a person may view a given act as ethical in one situation and as unethical in another.

Second, when we state that someone's behavior is unethical or immoral, we may mean that it is *reputed* to be unethical or immoral. Here we are accepting someone else's value judgment. We are implicitly assuming that another's internal standard for what is fair, right, or good is the same as ours, which may or may not be true. The situation in some instances is even more uncertain because the judgment being communicated is based not on the experience of the person communicating it but on that of someone else. The person is merely reporting what he or she was told.

The *natural law* tradition (see Chapter 2) is the primary avenue through which ethics influence Western legal thought (see Figure 2.1). Although philosophers are not in full agreement about what constitutes natural law, there are some common elements in the ways that they view it. According to Brody,

> what they have in common is the belief in a body of laws governing all people at all times and in a source for those laws other than the customs and institutions of a given society. Such beliefs are frequently accompanied by the additional beliefs that *no societies are authorized to create laws that conflict directly with natural laws, and that such conflicting laws may therefore be invalid* [italics mine]. In short, the natural law tradition asserts the

existence of a set of laws whose status as laws is based on their moral status (Brody, 1978, pp. 817–818).

Hence, we use our concept of what is ethical, or moral, both as a standard for assessing the fairness of existing laws and as a guide when encouraging legislators through lobbying (see Chapter 12) to enact new laws. If the majority of the voters in a political unit (a municipality, state, or country) regard an existing law as unfair, they may be able to have it removed by a legislative act. Of if a vocal minority of the voters in a political unit regard an existing situation as unfair, they may be able to convince the members of the appropriate legislature of this unfairness, which may motivate them to pass a law which would at least partially rectify the situation. Parents groups have used this mechanism to motivate legislatures to pass laws that provide appropriate special education, including speech-language pathology and audiology services, for handicapped children. And advocates for the deaf and severely speech impaired have used it to motivate legislatures to pass laws that provide them with "functionally equivalent" access to telephone communication by mandating and funding telecommunication relay services (Seelman, 1991).

Thus far in this discussion, ethics has been viewed as a *shaper of law*. The relationship between ethics and law can also be viewed in another way. From this second perspective it can be argued that *ethics is law* — in fact, the *highest* level of law. Hence, it follows that laws enacted by government should not be obeyed if obeying them would result in acts that are immoral—that is, contrary to natural law. Such laws, because they violate natural law, are regarded as *invalid*. One can, in fact, be punished by a court for obeying them. This actually occurred at the Nuremberg trials following World War II. A number of persons in postwar Germany were tried for genocide and convicted. It was argued at these trials that laws causing the Holocaust violated natural law and, hence, should not have been obeyed. Of course, refusing to obey a law because it violates one's sense of fairness may not be accepted as adequate justification by a court. (For further information about the relationship between ethics and law, see the article by Brody, 1978, in the *Encyclopedia of Bioethics*.)

ETHICS AND THE CLINICIAN

Ethical considerations impose restrictions and obligations on the professional activities of a clinician, both those associated with the *delivery of clinical services* and those associated with *clinical research*. These are imposed in two ways. The first is through the ethical values that all of us began to learn as children and that govern all aspects of our functioning. Some of these are likely to be associated with the Judeo-Christian tradition. And the second is through a *code of professional ethics* (or codes of professional ethics) that the clinician agreed to accept. He or she may have agreed to accept such a code because doing so was a requirement for certification or licensure. If this were the reason, failure to abide by the code could result in loss of certification or licensure (see Miller, 1983; Miller & Lubinski, 1986, for information concerning the types of unethical practices that have resulted in such a loss for speech-language pathologists and audiologists).

We will consider in this section the roles played by codes of professional ethics in regulating clinical functioning. The intent is to provide a *philosophical perspective* that should help speech-language pathologists and audiologists to better understand the function of the Code of Ethics of the American Speech-Language-Hearing Association as well as that of other professional ethical codes they are asked to accept.

Ethical considerations have been of concern to clinicians for at least the past two thousand years (Konold, 1978). Until the nineteenth century almost all clinicians were physicians, and they regarded the prevention and treatment of communicative disorders to be a part of their clinical responsibility. (Some physicians, particular those living in Europe who have had a residency in otolaryngology with a sub-specialty in *phoniatrics*, still view this as a part of their clinical responsibility.) Since the codes of ethics of almost all nonmedical clinical professions (including speech-language pathology and audiology) were based to some extent on codes of medical ethics, much can be learned about ethical aspects of clinical practice by studying the rationales for certain restrictions on the functioning of a physician that are imposed by medical ethical codes and their precursors—oaths and prayers.

Oaths and Prayers

Many of the restrictions and obligations mentioned in medical ethical codes have their origins in ancient prayers and oaths, particularly the latter. The *Daily Prayer of a Physician,* for example, which is one of the better known of the older statements on medical ethics, includes the following:

> Do not allow thirst for profit, ambition for renown and admiration, to interfere with my profession, for these are the enemies of truth and of love for mankind and they can lead astray in the great task of attending to the welfare of Thy creatures. Preserve the strength of my body and of my soul that they ever be ready to cheerfully help and support rich and poor, good and bad, enemy as well as friend. In the sufferer let me see only the human being. Illumine my mind that it recognize what presents itself and it may comprehend what is absent or hidden. . . . Let me never be absent-minded. May no strange thoughts divert my attention at the bedside of the sick, or disturb my mind in its silent labors, for great and sacred are the thoughtful deliberations required to preserve the . . . health of Thy creatures (Friedenwald, 1917, pp. 260–261).

The notion that a clinician needs to "hold paramount the welfare of persons served professionally," which is incorporated into all health care profession ethical codes in some form is acknowledged in this prayer. The ethical content of this excerpt, incidentally, would appear to be as relevant for speech-language pathologists and audiologists as it is for physicians.

Several of the restrictions and obligations that are mentioned in medical ethical codes also are alluded to in medical oaths. The following excerpt from the *Oath of Hippocrates,* which is thought to have been formulated more than two thousand years ago, is representative.

> I will apply dietitic measures for the benefit of the sick according to my ability and judgment; I will keep them from harm and injustice.
>
> I will neither give a deadly drug to anybody if asked for it nor will I make a suggestion to this effect. Similarly I will not give a woman an abortive remedy. In purity and holiness I will guard my life and my art.
>
> I will not use the knife, not even on sufferers from stone, but will withdraw in favor of such men as are engaged in this work.
>
> Whatever house I may visit, I will come for the benefit of the sick, remaining free of all intentional injustices, of all mischief and in particular of sexual relations with both female and male persons, be they free or slave.
>
> What I may see or hear in the course of the treatment or even outside of the treatment in regard to the life of men, which on no account one must

spread abroad, I will keep to myself holding such things shameful to be spoken about. (Edelstein, 1953, p. 3)

The five paragraphs in this excerpt allude to the ethical principle of "holding paramount the welfare of persons served professionally." A pledge is made in the first to use one's clinical skills in a manner likely to benefit one's patients in socially acceptable ways. In the second a pledge is made not to use one's skills to change a patient in socially unacceptable ways, even if asked to do so by the patient. Abortion apparently was socially unacceptable when this oath was formulated. During the twentieth century, it has been socially acceptable at times under certain circumstances. For this reason, contemporary codes of medical ethics do not forbid physicians to perform abortions under all circumstances. This illustrates an important aspect of professional ethics: What is ethical is not absolute, or unchangeable. An act that may be viewed as unethical at one point in time may not be viewed so at another.

A pledge is made in the third paragraph of the oath to make referrals to other professionals when this is needed to provide the patient with the best service possible. One implication of this pledge is that one should not attempt to provide services for which one has been inadequately trained or for which one is not licensed or certified. Physicians were not trained to be surgeons when the *Hippocratic Oath* was formulated: The practice of surgery was a separate profession. Since all of today's physicians are trained to do some surgery, this ethical prohibition is no longer enforced. This further illustrates the point that ethical precepts are not absolute, or unchangeable.

A pledge is made in the fourth paragraph of the oath to refrain from intentionally doing anything while functioning clinically that will be detrimental to the patient, regardless of his or her status (e.g., socioeconomic). This prohibition has relevance for clinical medical research that has been done on poor people without their knowledge or consent (e.g., the syphilis study that was conducted in the U.S. during the early part of this century in which a number of poor people who had the disease were not treated so that more could be learned about the types of damage it produces). And in the fifth, a pledge is made to not reveal what one has learned about a patient or his or her family to unauthorized persons. This precept—i.e., confidentiality—is present in some form in all health care profession ethical codes.

Codes of Ethics

While oaths and prayers can have a significant impact on the ethical behavior of those who subscribe to or use them, they are difficult to enforce. The restrictions and obligations that they place on the activities of practitioners are not usually described specifically enough for violations to be established beyond reasonable doubt. Practitioners may be able to claim with some justification that they did not realize that what they did constituted a violation of professional ethics. For this reason and several others, the format currently used in medicine and other health care professions for presenting ethical precepts is the code of ethics.

The broad ethical concerns addressed in the codes of ethics of most health care professions tend to be quite similar. The results of a survey conducted under the auspices of Georgetown University's Kennedy Institute and the *Encyclopedia of Bioethics* Project of 525 organizations representing a cross section of the health care professions suggests that the typical code exhorts practitioners

> ... to preserve human life, to be a good citizen, to prevent the exploitation of patients, to promote the highest quality health care available, to perform their duties with objectivity and accuracy, to strive for professional excellence through continuing education, to avoid discriminatory practices, to promote the interest and ideals of the profession, to expose unethical and incompetent colleagues, to encourage public health through health-care education, to render service at times of public emergencies, to promote harmonious relations with other health-care professions, and to protect the welfare, dignity, and confidentiality of patients (Gass, 1978, p. 1725).

The typical code also provides practitioners with ethical guidelines that address such practical issues relevant to clinical functioning as " ... advertising, billing procedures, self-aggrandizement [i.e., making oneself appear more knowledgeable and competent than one is], conflicts of interest, professional courtesy, public and media relations, employment and supervision of auxiliary personnel, use of secret remedies and exclusive methods, as well as the location and physical appearance of the office practice" (Gass, 1978, pp. 1725–1726).

It should be apparent from this brief overview that the typical health care profession code of ethics contains guidelines and precepts that address most aspects of clinical practice. The remainder of this section is devoted to an examination of several of these that are particularly relevant to clinical functioning in speech-language pathology and audiology. The order in which they are discussed does not necessarily reflect their importance.

Confidentiality. One of the most fundamental of all the ethical precepts is the need for confidentiality in the relationship between client and clinician. This need was recognized early in medical ethical thinking as evidenced by its inclusion in the *Oath of Hippocrates.* Originally, this requirement was absolute. Anything that a patient told a physician was supposed to be regarded as confidential and not to be revealed to anyone without the patient's permission. In fact, if a patient told a physician that he or she was going to murder someone, it would have been regarded as unethical for the physician to inform the authorities. Judging by contemporary medical ethical codes (a representative sample of which are included in the appendix of the *Encyclopedia of Bioethics*), this requirement is no longer regarded as absolute. Information obtained from a patient can be revealed without permission under certain circumstances. The American Medical Association's Principles of Medical Ethics, formulated in 1957 and revised in 1971 (Reich, 1978, pp. 1750–1754), for example, specified three circumstances under which it would not be regarded as unethical to reveal information obtained from a patient without first securing the patient's permission.

> A physician may not reveal the confidences entrusted to him in the course of medical attendance, or the deficiencies he may observe in the character of patients, *unless he is required to do so by law or unless it becomes necessary in order to protect the welfare of the individual or of the community* [italics mine].

These same three exceptions, incidentally, were mentioned in the current (1991) Code of Ethics of the American Speech-Language-Hearing Association.

The first of these exceptions—being required *by law* to reveal information without the patient's permission—is the one that speech-language pathologists and audiologists are likely to encounter most frequently. Either a civil or criminal court can order them to reveal such information. The likelihood that they could successfully refuse to reveal information requested by a court because they view it as *privileged communication* would depend on the precedents that govern the decisions of the court issuing the order. If a court previously had allowed similar information obtained under similar circumstances to be regarded as privileged communication, it may be willing to do so again. You should consult an attorney to determine the likelihood that a court will honor your refusal to reveal certain information because you regard it as privileged communication.

The second of these exceptions—to protect the welfare of the individual—is apt to be a difficult one to justify. In fact, a clinician would have to assume the *burden of proof* to justify revealing information about a patient without the patient's permission because he or she thought that doing so would protect the patient's welfare. Revealing such information could result in a clinician's being sued by the patient as well as being charged with violating professional ethics. A speech-language pathologist or audiologist would be faced with this type of ethical dilemma when deciding whether to reveal information acquired from a child client to the child's parents. Aside from possible legal and ethical consequences of revealing information about a client without permission, doing so would be likely to have a negative impact on your relationship with the client. He or she may no longer be willing to trust you.

The third of these exceptions—to protect the welfare of the community—is apt to be extremely difficult to justify. About the only circumstance under which it would be relatively simple for a clinician to do so would be if a client revealed that he or she was planning to commit a crime. A clinician might with some justification feel an obligation to the community to inform the appropriate authorities.

The confidentiality precept applies to both oral and written communication between client and clinician and includes reports and other clinical records. Information in a client's clinic folder and/or in his or her computer database file(s) should be regarded as confidential, and it ordinarily would be regarded as unethical to release it without his or her permission. It also could be breaking the law to do so. Legal-ethical aspects of clinical records management are discussed in Chapter 7.

Improvement of Clinical Knowledge and Skills. One precept mentioned in all health care profession codes of ethics is "holding paramount the welfare of persons served professionally." This implies that the clinician will use the most effective therapy approaches (intervention strategies) that the state of the art will allow. The American Medical Association in its Principles of Medical Ethics states that "Physicians should strive continually to improve medical knowledge and skill, and should make available to their patients and colleagues the benefits of their professional attainments." This precept, by implication, places several obligations on a clinician. First is an obligation to keep up to date by reading professional journals, attending workshops and conventions, and taking courses (including continuing education ones). The more knowledge-able clinicians are about the state of the art in clinical knowledge and technique, the more effective they are likely to be when attempting to ameliorate their client's problems. Hence, a failure to keep up to date is a serious violation of professional ethics because it is incompatible with holding paramount the welfare of one's clients (Carney, 1991).

A second obligation implied by this precept is for the clinician to evaluate his or her intervention strategies to determine their effectiveness. Doing so would tend to increase effectiveness as a clinician, assuming that intervention strategies which were not having the desired impacts on clients would be modified or discarded. For further discussion about the need for clinicians to do therapy outcome research, see Chapter 2 in *Research Design and Evaluation in Speech-Language Pathology and Audiology* (Silverman, 1993).

A third obligation that this ethical precept appears to require a clinician to accept is to advance clinical knowledge and techniques, if he or she has the opportunity. By doing so clinicians have an opportunity to improve not only their own effectiveness, but also that of other clinicians (see Chapter 2 in Silverman, 1993). One way by which clinicians have met this responsibility is by reporting the impacts of therapy programs—both positive and negative—that they have used with patients (while, of course, maintaining the patients' anonymity).

Truth-Telling and Informed Consent. A clinician has an obligation to be honest with patients about the nature of their condition, the prognosis for improvement, and the probable impacts (both positive and negative) of the possible therapy approaches, unless receipt of such information is likely to be detrimental to them. A clinician may also have a similar obligation to the families of patients, particularly when patients are children or severely impaired adults who are unable to understand the information or on whom such information is likely to have a detrimental effect. The ethical ramifications of telling the truth have been dealt with extensively in the medical literature, particularly with regard to the desirability of informing a patient that he or she is dying. The arguments that have been advanced for truth-telling, both pro and con, have implications beyond this context and, hence, are summarized in this section.

One of the main arguments in favor of truth-telling is that a patient has the right to decide whether he or she wishes to participate in the intervention program recommended by the clinician. Unless a patient has been provided with accurate information about the nature of the condition, its prognosis, and probably impacts (both positive and negative) of the recommended intervention program (or alternative intervention programs), the patient's consent to participate in the program is not likely to be viewed by a court as legally binding. If a patient is given such information, a court is likely to regard the consent as constituting *informed consent*. The assumption, of course, is being made that the patient can understand the information presented—that is, it is being assumed that the patient does not have a neurological condition such as receptive aphasia, mental retardation, Alzheimer's disease, or cerebral arteriosclerosis; or a hearing loss; or difficulty comprehending English because it is a second language. It is also being assumed that the patient is not a young child.

One of the main arguments against truth-telling, especially complete truth-telling, is that it can have a detrimental effect on the patient. If a patient is told the prognosis for improvement is poor, the therapy may be less beneficial than it would have been if the patient had been given a less truthful or less complete statement of prognosis. Having been given a poor prognosis, a patient may reject therapy or become so despondent that he or she cannot benefit maximally from it.

This situation illustrates a type of ethical dilemma that we frequently confront—one with two possible courses of action, either of which can result in our violating an ethical principle. If a patient is given an honest statement of prognosis, it may have a detrimental effect, thus violating the ethical principle that the welfare of persons served professionally must be paramount. On the other hand, if a patient is not given a truthful statement of prognosis because such a statement would be likely to have a detrimental effect, this would violate the ethical principle that a clinician should be truthful with patients. Confronted by such a situation, a clinician has to *weigh the competing ethical considerations* to determine which is (or are) the most important.

One aspect of truth-telling that is mentioned in a number of health care profession codes of ethics is not guaranteeing cures. Many variables can influence how much a patient will improve, and a clinician can rarely predict their impacts with accuracy.

Informed consent is an important ethical consideration not only when providing clinical services but also when doing *clinical research*. Individuals should be fully informed about potential risks when they are asked to participate in a research project. This topic is discussed in Chapter 10.

Not Exploiting Persons Served Professionally. Most, if not all, health care profession codes of ethics implicitly or explicitly prohibit practitioners from exploiting those whom they are serving professionally. Such exploitation can arise from several sources. One is fees charged for services rendered. The American Medical Association's Principles of Medical Ethics, for example, includes the following statement:

> In the practice of medicine a physician should limit the source of his professional income to medical services actually rendered by him, or under his supervision, to his patients. His fee should be commensurate with the services rendered and the patient's ability to pay. He should neither pay or receive a commission for referral of patients. Drugs, remedies, or appliances may be dispensed or supplied by the physician provided it is in the best interests of the patient.

Hence, a practitioner would be exploiting those whom he or she is serving professionally by charging fees that are higher than would be commensurate with the services he or she rendered and their ability to pay. He or she would also be exploiting them by paying or receiving a commission for referring them to other practitioners, by selling them things they do not need, or for charging them for services not rendered.

A second source of such exploitation is accepting patients for treatment or continuing treatment when the prognosis for improvement (or further improvement) is extremely poor. Private practitioners are particularly likely to be tempted to do this if their caseloads are relatively small and discharging or refusing patients will result in a loss of income. By rendering services to such patients practitioners will also be exploiting society if the fees charged for serving them are being paid (partially or completely) by a third party, such as an insurance program.

Monitoring Compliance with the Code of Ethics. Many health care profession codes of ethics require practitioners to report code violations to the board that monitors compliance with it and to cooperate with this board when its members are investigating the ethical behavior of fellow practitioners. The following statement from the American Medical Association's Principles of Medical Ethics is representative:

> The medical profession should safeguard the public and itself against physicians deficient in moral character or professional competence. Physicians should observe all laws, uphold the dignity and honor of the

profession and its self-imposed disciplines. They should expose, without hesitation, illegal or unethical conduct of fellow members of the profession.

This obligation is a logical consequence of accepting what is probably the most fundamental of these ethical principles—holding paramount the welfare of persons served professionally. The persons whose welfare you are obliged to hold paramount include not only those with whom you work personally but also those who are served by other members of your profession (Koenigsknecht, 1990a). For speech-language pathologists and audiologists, this would include all communicatively handicapped persons who are, have been, or could be consumers of their services (see Koenigsknecht, 1990c; National forum on consumer rights, 1990). Thus, holding paramount the welfare of persons served by members of your profession obliges you to expose the unethical conduct and incompetence of fellow professionals. Of course, if you charge a fellow professional with being unethical or incompetent, you must either be prepared to prove it or to provide sufficient evidence to justify an investigation. Otherwise, you may find yourself the defendant in a defamation suit.

Patient Selection and Discrimination. To what extent is it permissible for clinicians to choose whom they will and will not serve? Is it always unethical to consider race, religion, sex, and ability to pay? Is it unethical to exclude from ones caseload persons who have a particular disease—e.g., AIDS? These questions are answered somewhat differently in the various health care profession codes of ethics. In some, such as the American Medical Association's Principles of Ethics, they are dealt with directly and the clinician is allowed considerable freedom in patient selection:

A physician may choose whom he will serve. In an emergency, however, he should render service to the best of his ability.

In others, such as the American Psychological Association's Ethical Standards for Psychologists (Reich, 1978, pp. 1811–1815), they are dealt with indirectly, if at all. And in still others, such as the 1991 Code of Ethics of the American Speech-Language-Hearing Association (see Appendix D), they are dealt with directly and clinicians are prohibited from discriminating against clients on certain bases:

Individuals must not discriminate in the delivery of professional services on any basis that is unjustifiable or irrelevant to the need for and potential benefit from such services, such as race, sex, age, religion, national origin, sexual orientation, or handicapping condition.

There is one area of possible discrimination that does not currently appear to be addressed directly in many health care profession codes of ethics that we will consider here. This is choosing not to provide services (or to provide only limited services) to persons whose bills are paid by some third parties, such as governmental insurance programs (e.g., Medicare and Medicaid). The fees they pay for certain services are sometimes considerably lower than those usually charged for them, and providing services to those covered by such programs tends to entail a relatively large amount of paperwork. Also, the agencies responsible for administering these programs may be relatively slow in paying, which can cause cash-flow problems. This issue is addressed indirectly in some health care profession codes of ethics: The American Medical Association in its Principles of Medical Ethics, for example, states that fees charged "should be commensurate with . . . the patient's ability to pay." This statement would appear to imply that a patient should not be denied services because the fees that the patient can be charged are lower than the practitioner's usual ones. The ethical issues here are murky, and clinicians will have to rely on their own sense of what is fair or on the fee policies of their employers when deciding whether to serve such patients.

Advertising. Most health care profession codes of ethics place some restrictions on the advertising of clinical services, but not as many as previously. The first Code of Ethics of the American Medical Association (1947), which served as the model for subsequent health care profession codes of ethics in the United States, placed the following restrictions on the advertising of such services:

> It is derogatory to the dignity of the profession, to resort to public advertisement or private cards or handbills, inviting the attention of individuals affected with particular diseases—publicly offering advice and medicine to the poor gratis, or promising radical cures; to publish cases and operations in the daily prints, or suffer such publications to be made;—to invite laymen to be present at operations—to boast of cures and remedies—to adduce certificates of skill and success, or to perform any similar acts. These are the ordinary practices of empirics [charlatans and quacks], and are highly reprehensible to a regular physician (Reich, 1978, pp. 1741–1742).

It would appear from this excerpt that the original impetus for restricting advertising was to differentiate the trained practitioner from the charlatan or quack (Ciuccio, 1990). (The term *quack*, as used here, refers to a practitioner who lacks the qualifications and training regarded as necessary by proponents of the profession's licensure and certification requirements. There have been at least a few cases in which a practitioner who was viewed as a *quack* was later viewed as an *innovator.*)

Restrictions on the advertising of clinical services have been relaxed somewhat during the past twenty years (Ciuccio, 1990). There appear to be several reasons why these restrictions were relaxed. First, there is an obvious need to make people aware of who is a qualified practitioner. If only unqualified practitioners are permitted to advertise their services, the public will have difficulty locating qualified ones. Thus, physicians and other health care professionals (including speech-language pathologists and audiologists) were permitted to list themselves under appropriate headings in the *Yellow Pages* of the telephone book and to discreetly inform both the public and professionals in the community who may serve as referral sources about their services. In some health care fields (e.g., medicine) restrictions on advertising have been relaxed to the point where it is no longer regarded as unethical for practitioners to advertise their services on television.

A second reason for relaxing restrictions on advertising is that such restrictions have been viewed by the courts as constituting *restraint of trade* (Ciuccio, 1990). From this perspective, restrictions on advertising keep costs to consumers high by eliminating competition among practitioners. If practitioners were to directly or indirectly advertise the costs of their services, consumers probably would consider cost when selecting a practitioner. Hence, practitioners would have some motivation to keep their fees reasonable, which, at least theoretically, would tend to lower costs to consumers. Since the advertising of fees for professional services is a relatively recent phenomenon, it is uncertain how much impact it actually will have on the costs of such services.

For additional information about ethical issues in clinical/professional practice, see *Casebook on Ethical Principles for Psychologists* (1987), Flower (1986), McDowell (1991), Rosner & Weinstock (1990), and Wood (1986).

CODE OF ETHICS OF THE
AMERICAN SPEECH-LANGUAGE-HEARING ASSOCIATION

The Code of Ethics of the American Speech-Language-Hearing Association (ASHA) has much in common with those of other health care professions. It imposes on speech-language pathologists and audiologists all of the restrictions and obligations that have been discussed in this chapter. And like the others, it has evolved considerably since its initial formulation (see Appendix D and LC amends Code of Ethics, 1990) and will most likely continue to evolve as the law changes and as speech-language pathologists and audiologists are called upon to meet new challenges.

The membership of ASHA has been concerned with ethical issues since the founding of the Association in 1925. In fact, one of the reasons mentioned for founding the organization, according to Paden, was "To establish scientific standards and *codes of ethics* [italics mine]" (1970, p. 73). The relatively high level of concern that the founders of ASHA had about professional ethics was, at least in part, a reaction to the unprofessional conduct of some practitioners who treated speech disorders, especially stuttering.

> Such persons were known, for example, to make rash guarantees of cure, to require their patients to sign statements that they would never reveal their methods, to charge exorbitant fees, and to otherwise degrade the image of the profession (Paden, 1970, p. 73).

Also, a few were known to treat speech disorders completely or almost completely by correspondence. Many of the practices that were prohibited in the various revisions of the ASHA ethical code (see Appendix D) were a part of the modus operandi of some nineteenth- and twentieth-century practitioners.

The primary ethical focus during the early years of ASHA seemed to be on preventing unethical practitioners from joining rather than on monitoring the ethical practices of members. This may partially explain why, prior to 1950, association statements about ethics were included in the section of the association's constitution that dealt with membership requirements rather than in a separate document. This focus also is evident from the qualifications for membership that were included in the original (1926) constitution of the association. There were five qualifications listed, one of which was the following:

> Possession of a professional reputation untainted by a past record (or a present record) of unethical practices such as blatant commercialization of professional services, or guaranteeing of "cures" for stated sums of money.

It apparently was not until the early 1940s that the association was called upon to investigate a complaint about the ethical practices of a member

(Paden, 1970). (For further information about the early development of the ASHA Code of Ethics, see Paden, 1970.)

The primary ethical focus of ASHA at the present time (as it seems to have been since the 1950s) is on monitoring the ethical practices of its members. All members who are engaged in clinical practice and all nonmembers who have ASHA clinical certification are required to agree to be bound by the Code of Ethics. The change in focus from admission to membership to monitoring of membership appears to have come about largely because most persons who joined ASHA after the 1940s had not had sufficient paid clinical experience for their ethical standards to be assessed. Most of those who sought membership during the early years had been functioning as practitioners for a significant period of time, which made it possible to assess their ethical standards prior to admitting them to membership.

The issues addressed in the various revisions of the ASHA Code (see Appendix D) parallel those addressed in other health care profession codes of ethics at the same points in time. This has occurred because the health care professions have had to cope with similar ethical problems during given time periods. During the 1970s, for example, a number of these professions had to cope with ethical problems associated with their practitioners' treating patients whose therapy is paid for by a *third party*, such as Medicare or Medicaid. Most of the ethical issues that are addressed in the ASHA Code are discussed elsewhere in this chapter.

Codes of ethics deal with *general principles of ethical behavior*. The application of these general principles to specific situations encountered by clinicians often requires some interpretation. A series of articles has appeared in ASHA publications over the years (mostly in the journal *Asha*), some with titles beginning *Issues in Ethics*, that have attempted to interpret how the ASHA Code can be applied to certain situations encountered by clinicians, including the following: *third-party payment* (Bangs, 1970); *dispensing of products* (Ethical practices board interpretations on principles governing the dispensing of products to persons with communicative disorders, 1976); *speech-language pathologists doing myofunctional therapy* (EPB interpretations of "Joint Committee Statement on Tongue Thrust," 1975); *advertising of members' products* (Issues in ethics: Advertising of members' products, 1974); *honoring of contracts* (Issues in ethical practice—Responsibilities concerning the honoring of a verbal or written contract, 1958); *fees for clinical services provided by students* (Issues in ethics: Fees for clinical services provided by students, 1978);

action by ASHA for violation of state association or licensure ethical codes (Issues in ethics—Ethical practice inquiries: State versus ASHA decision differences, 1978); *speech-language pathologists functioning as audiologists and vice versa* (Issues in ethics: Clinical practice by members in the area in which they are not certified, 1977; Issues in Ethics: Clinical practice by certificate holders in areas in which they are not certified, 1986); *CFY supervisors' responsibilities* (Issues in ethics: CFY supervisors' responsibilities, 1980a); *degrees from "diploma mills"* (Issues in ethics: The bogus degree, 1974); *use of supportive personnel* (Issues in ethics: ASHA policy re: supportive personnel, 1979); *public statements and announcements by members* (Issues in ethics: Public statements and general announcements: Guidelines and procedures, 1977; Issues in ethics: Public announcements and public statements, 1981); *ASHA members who are uncertified engaging in clinical practice* (Issues in ethics: Identification of members engaged in clinical practice without certification, 1973), *listing in telephone directories* (Issues in ethics: Guidelines for telephone directories, 1974); *gratuities* (Issues in ethics: Gratuities, 1978); *augmentative communication* (Nonspeech communication: A position paper, 1980); *private practice* (Issues in Ethics: Drawing cases for private practice from primary place of employment, 1980b); *research* (Issues in Ethics: Ethics in research and professional practice, 1982); *use of graduate degrees* (Issues in Ethics: Use of graduate degrees by members and/or certificate holders, 1987); *competition* (Issues in Ethics: Competition, 1989a); *prescription* (Issues in Ethics: Prescription, 1989b); and *supervision of student clinicians* (Issues in Ethics: Supervision of student clinicians, 1991).

While the ASHA Code of Ethics provides guidelines for dealing with most situations a speech-language pathologist or audiologist is likely to encounter, it does not do so for all of them. For example, consider the following scenario: A speech-language pathologist after being hired to supervise a public school system clinical service program discovers that there are two or three staff members at the BA level offering direct services. The state views these persons as qualified, but ASHA doesn't agree. How should he or she handle the situation?

The *Ethical Practice Board* (EPB) is responsible for investigating charges of code violations by ASHA members (see Ethical Practice Board statement of practices and procedures, 1991). If the preponderance of evidence following a careful investigation suggests that the member did violate the Code of Ethics, the board can recommend that disciplinary action of some kind be taken. The most extreme action that it can recommend is revocation of membership and certification (see *Actions of the Ethical Practice Board,* 1986, 1988, 1989a, 1989b, 1991a, 1991b, 1991c). Information about procedures for filing or answering a complaint can be obtained from the ASHA national office. Anyone who has been accused of violating the ASHA Code and is being investigated by EPB would probably be wise to consult with an attorney.

Chapter IV

LICENSURE, CERTIFICATION, REGISTRATION, AND ACCREDITATION

O ne of the ways by which our legal system directly and indirectly influences the clinical functioning of speech-language pathologists and audiologists is through the mechanisms of licensure, certification, registration and accreditation. These set limits on the *client populations* to whom a person certified or licensed as a speech-language pathologist or audiologist may provide services and on the *services* that he or she may provide to persons in these populations. A person certified or licensed as an audiologist would be permitted to provide certain services to certain populations (e.g., fitting hearing aids to persons who have hearing losses) that a person certified or licensed as a speech-language pathologist ordinarily would not be permitted to provide and vice versa. Licensure and certification also set limits on *how services can be provided* by requiring adherence to a code of ethics. Failure to function in a manner consistent with the code of ethics can result in one's license being revoked or one's certification being taken away (see Actions of the Ethical Practices Board, 1986, 1988, 1989a, 1989b, 1991). In addition, licensure and certification impose restrictions on how practitioners are *trained*. The requirements for the Certificates of Clinical Competence in Speech-Language Pathology and Audiology awarded by the American Speech-Language-Hearing Association and state licensure (including that for the public schools) influence the curriculums of speech-language pathology and audiology training programs. Finally, licensure and certification requirements can influence how speech-language pathologists and audiologists are *paid for their services*. Some health insurance programs (e.g., Medicare) stipulate that for speech-language pathology services to be covered they must be provided by a practitioner who has met the requirements for A.S.H.A. Certification or an appropriate license issued by the state. Also, if a school district wishes to be at least partially reimbursed by the state for services to communicatively handicapped children, they must be provided by speech-language pathologists who are credentialed by the state department of public instruction.

WHAT IS THE MOTIVATION FOR INITIATING LICENSURE, CERTIFICATION, REGISTRATION AND ACCREDITATION?

Whenever individuals or groups decide to attempt to change the status quo, it is almost always because they expect to derive some benefit from doing so. Their expectations may or may not be realistic. But so long as they believe they will benefit from a change, they are likely to attempt to bring it about. The reason or reasons they give for wanting to change the status quo may not be the real reasons or may not be all of them. Rather, they are apt to be reasons they feel would be *acceptable* to those who must approve the change.

The regulation of professionals through licensure, certification, accreditation, and registration in the United States is a relatively recent phenomenon historically. In the health field it appears to have begun with medicine. Prior to 1800 many states attempted to regulate medical practice with varying degrees of success. It was not until just before the civil war, however, that interest in regulating health professionals reached a national level with the establishment of the American Medical Association in 1847 and the American Dental Association in 1859 (Levine, 1978). Practitioners in most other health-related fields (including speech-language pathology and audiology) were not regulated prior to the twentieth century.

The individuals and groups who seek regulation for an occupation (particularly a profession) tend to be those who are members of it rather than consumers of its services. The investment required for achieving some form of regulation is usually substantial—with regard to both time and money. Since regulation would be expected to place restrictions on the activities of those seeking it, why would they be motivated to pursue it? What *benefits* would they expect to receive from achieving it? My intent in this section is to provide at least a partial answer to these questions.

The primary justification that usually is given for regulating an occupation is the *protection of public health, safety, or morals* (see Lynch, 1986, for a discussion of this justification as it applies to our field). Those seeking regulation argue that without it, incompetent practitioners will offer their services. Prospective buyers of these services are said not to be able to distinguish between qualified and unqualified persons, and this is considered to be especially true if consumers buy services of the particular kind only at infrequent intervals. Where the consequences of the employment of unqualified persons can be expected to be seriously adversive to the purchaser, and especially where the consequences of incompetently rendered service are irreversible, it is thought to be desirable that ... some examining or other procedure [be administered] to determine who are qualified to practice, and prevent those who are unqualified from offering their services. The average quality of those permitted to practice is raised, and by exclusion of "quacks" and incompetents the public is protected from the error of employing them (Rottenberg, 1968, p. 283).

Though these arguments were formulated to justify licensing, they have been used to justify other forms of regulation as well.

Although regulation can be justified on the basis that it tends to *raise the average quality* of the services offered by the members of a profession, this may not be the primary reason why they are motivated to pursue it. Their primary reason may be to gain *legal status,* or recognition, for the profession:

Once a profession is awarded legal status and is given the exclusive right to practice in the field of its competence, it can inhibit the practice of imposters by taking action in the courts. ... Each profession defines an area of practice in which it has a monopoly and fights hard to preserve that unique area (Lum, 1978, p. 156).

Thus, by gaining legal status through regulation a health profession can establish what its members hope will be an *exclusive claim to a segment of the health service territory.* The total territory consists of all services for preventing and ameliorating all the disorders that a person can develop; each profession is seeking to be granted the exclusive right to provide *certain* of these services to those who have *certain* disorders. If they are successful, they will have a monopoly (or close to a monopoly) on the delivery of certain services to the segment of the territory to which they have staked a claim. Medicine is an example of a profession that has been successful in establishing a near monopoly on the delivery of certain services to a segment of this territory.

When a profession is awarded a monopoly, or near monopoly, for the delivery of certain services, it is expected to see to it that these services are provided in a responsible manner. According to Lum,

Society accords a monopoly to a profession with respect to its practice and standard setting on the premise that no lay person understands esoteric knowledge on which the profession rests, and therefore no lay person can judge what should be done. Society allows a profession to hold a monopoly because it is convinced that the profession is dedicated to an ethical or altruistic ideal in serving society. Society continues to allow this monopoly as long as it is convinced that a profession is exercising its privileges responsibly and aids and/or serves its clientele without exploitation.

Under its monopoly, a profession has the purpose of protecting not only the society it serves, but also its members, making it possible for them to practice effectively. Its protection, which occurs through methods passed on by socialization, takes different form as the profession confronts internal as well as external dangers.

Internally, a profession must protect society and its members against the incompetent or dishonest member whose actions may damage trust in the profession. A profession controls the number and kinds of persons who are allowed to enter and to study through the establishment of admission criteria and determining the length and types of programs allowed. These controls are imposed in order to prevent incompetent persons from entering the profession and to avoid an oversupply of practitioners as well. In addition, it controls the body of knowledge on which the practice rests and maintains the quality and standards of its education through a process of external accreditation. It further controls admission to the profession through licensing procedures as well as through various certification and credential procedures. It opposes efforts to establish conditions that would make its practice difficult or impossible. Each profession has an obligation to police its own ranks and make certain that those who wear the name and display the license are in fact ethical and competent practitioners. From this obligation stem efforts to enforce the code of ethics of the profession even to the extent of expelling members who flagrantly violate provisions of its code. Thus, a physician can have his [or her] license revoked and a lawyer can be "disbarred." Professional associations aid practitioners in obtaining legal sanction for their monopoly (Lum, 1978, pp. 155–156).

In a sense, when a profession is granted a monopoly, it enters into a *contract* with the community (through the legislature) that granted it. As compensation for the legal status accorded it, the members of the profession agree to provide certain services that are of an *acceptable quality.* If they fail to do what they promised, the community has the right (perhaps even the obligation) to terminate their monopoly as providers of these services.

One possible result of regulating the practice of a profession is reducing the number of persons entering it. The higher the cost to qualify as a practitioner, the less likely persons are to attempt to do so (particularly if they do not expect the financial rewards from qualifying to be worth the effort). Several factors are likely to contribute to the cost of entering a profession. The most obvious one is the cost of the training or education required for doing so. In addition to the direct cost associated with this education or training, there is also an indirect one—the money the person would have earned if he or she had worked instead of pursuing the necessary schooling.

Another cost associated with entering a profession is the investment of time and energy required to gain the knowledge and experience necessary to be licensed or certified. When the members of a professional group are proposing licensing or certification requirements, it is not uncommon for them to make these requirements *more demanding* than those they were required to satisfy, and if their recommendations are accepted, to award themselves the new (or revised) license or certificate through a *grandfather clause*. Such clauses stimulate "that those who have already entered and are practicing the occupation be qualified *pro forma* and exempted from examination" (Rottenberg, 1968, p. 283). The term *pro forma* in this context is used to suggest that the license or certificate is awarded not on the basis of a conviction that those awarded it under the grandfather clause are qualified, but merely to facilitate acceptance of the license or certificate by existing practitioners. A person would be unlikely to support a change in requirements for certification or licensure if its adoption means that he or she would no longer qualify for certification or licensure.

HOW ARE OCCUPATIONS REGULATED?

A number of approaches are used to regulate the entrance of new practitioners into an occupation (see Figure 4.1). Some are initiated and administered by a professional organization, and others are administered by a governmental agency (usually a state one). Each of these is described in this section.

Types of Regulation Administered by a Professional Organization

A professional organization can regulate the practice of an occupation in two main ways: through certification and accreditation. Both are used

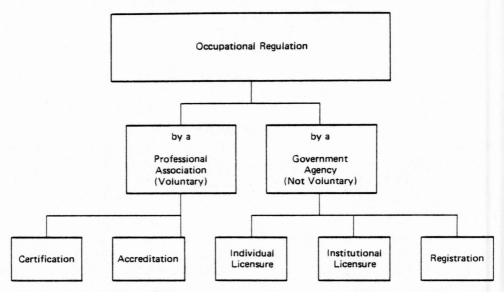

FIGURE 4.1 Approaches used for occupational regulation in health-related fields.

by the American Speech-Language-Hearing Association to regulate the practice of speech-language pathology and audiology.

Certification. Certification is "a voluntary mechanism by which a nongovernmental agency or association grants recognition to an individual who has met certain predetermined qualifications specified by that agency or association" (Roemer, 1974, p. 26). Because certification is a *voluntary* mechanism, persons who are not certified in an occupation can legally enter it (assuming that no license is required). They may, however, have difficulty finding employment because employers may refuse to hire those who do not possess the certification. There are several reasons. First, it simplifies the hiring process. The person doing the hiring can avoid having to evaluate the competency of each applicant by insisting on possession of the appropriate certification. Its possession by an applicant signifies to the employer that the applicant's education and experience have been adequate to meet at least minimum performance standards. Second, it may simplify the process for obtaining payment from *third parties* (such as private and government-sponsored insurance programs) for clinical services. [This also applied for licensure—see White, 1986.] Third parties stipulate that they will only pay for services that are provided by persons whom they regard as qualified practitioners. Almost all such providers would consider a person who was qualified as competent by the national association to which members of the profession belong to be a qualified practitioner. (An example of such an association would be the American Speech-Language-Hearing Association).

Certification may be offered to acknowledge either *basic* or *specialty* qualifications. When all states regulate the practice of a profession on a basic level through licensure (as is the case in medicine), then professional organizations tend to concentrate their efforts on *specialty certification*. (A specialty for which certification is offered in medicine is otolaryngology.) If in the future all states regulate the practice of speech-language pathology and audiology through licensure, the American Speech-Language-Hearing Association will be likely to emphasize specialty certification (e.g., in treating fluency disorders) rather than its present certification program (Governmental regulation, 1969).

Certification can be offered for a *relatively narrow* subject matter specialty, such as administering and interpreting a particular test or using a specific intervention approach. Tests that practitioners in the field of communicative disorders have been certified to administer and interpret include the *Porch Index of Communicative Ability* (Porch, 1967) and the *Staggered Spondaic Word Test* (Katz, Basil, & Smith, 1963). Intervention strategies that they have been certified to use include augmentative communication with Blissymbols (Kates, McNaughton, & Silverman, no date) and the *Hollins Precision Fluency Shaping Program* (Webster, 1974). While organizations that award this type of certification cannot legally prevent uncertified persons from using their tests or intervention strategies, they can make it difficult for them to do so by making full sets of materials available only to those who are certified or in the process of becoming certified.

Most professional certification programs have several components in addition to requiring acceptance of a code of ethics. First, they require the successful completion of one or more courses that many or may not be offered for academic credit by a college or university. Second, they usually require a specified minimum amount of supervised practical (practicum) experience. Third, they may require an "internship" following completion of the academic and practicum requirements. Fourth, they may require the passing of an examination. And fifth, they may require persons who have the certification to expose themselves periodically to continuing education. (The words *expose themselves* were used because most continuing education courses do not have examinations or other mechanisms for determining how much participants have learned.) The American Speech-Language-Hearing Association's Certificates of

Clinical Competence in Speech-Language Pathology and Audiology require the first four of these components. The fifth is encouraged through awarding of the ACE certificate.

While certification encourages practitioners to obtain the training necessary to perform their services competently and to behave ethically in their interactions with others, it has several limitations as a mechanism for insuring competence. According to Roemer,

> The basic requirement for certification is completion of an approved educational program, but the multiplicity of educational programs in different settings for the same occupation makes surveillance difficult. For many health occupations, no substitution of work experience or recognition of equivalent qualifications is allowed in place of academic qualifications for certification. Very few certifying bodies use examinations developed by professional testing agencies. [A.S.H.A. does use such examinations for its certification program.] In some cases, use of proficiency examinations might be a better measure of skills than written examinations. Not all certifying bodies require continuing quality of performance by persons certified, though they may require continuing membership in the association. (1974, p. 29)

Further discussion concerning the limitations of certification can be found in the *Proceedings of the 1971 Conference on Certification in Allied Health*, sponsored by the U.S. Department of Health, Education, and Welfare (DHEW Publication Number NIH 73-246, September, 1971).

Accreditation. A second approach that a professional organization can use for regulating the practice of an occupation is to *establish standards* for the curriculum and administration of programs that train new practitioners. Such programs may be offered by a college or university or by some other institution. (A hospital school of nursing would be an example of a professional training program that is offered by an institution other than a college or university.) By influencing the curriculums of programs that are training the practitioners for a profession, a professional organization can influence both the number of new persons who enter it and how they are trained.

A professional organization can influence the numbers of new practitioners entering a field in several ways by exercising control over curriculum. First, it can control the amount of education a person has to obtain before he or she is employable as a practitioner. The greater the amount beyond a certain level (e.g., a bachelor's degree), the fewer the number of persons who probably will be interested in entering the field, particularly if there are other fields offering similar rewards for which entrance is less costly. All else being equal, an occupation requiring a graduate degree for entrance probably would attract fewer people than one requiring a bachelor's degree.

By controlling curriculum a professional organization can influence the number of new practitioners entering a field in a second way: This is by limiting the number and size of training programs. It can make such programs sufficiently expensive to discourage some universities and colleges from beginning or continuing them. Or it can force training programs to limit their enrollments by establishing maximum acceptable faculty-student ratios.

By controlling curriculum a professional organization can obviously influence *how* practitioners are trained. It can influence the training not only of practitioners who will be certified as competent by it but of others as well. The American Speech-Language-Hearing Association through its accreditation program influences the training of students who will seek its Certificates of Clinical Competence as well as those who will not seek one of them—e.g., those who only will seek to be licensed by a state department of public instruction as a public school speech-language clinician.

What is accreditation and how does it function? Accreditation is "the process by which an agency or organization evaluates or recognizes a program of study or an institution as meeting certain predetermined qualifications or standards" (Standards for federal funding, 1972, p. 547). The agency or organization is not directly (or officially) affiliated with any municipal, state, or federal governmental unit. It may, however, be indirectly affiliated with one or more such units. One way by which this can occur is an agency or organization being officially recognized by a governmental unit as the regional or national accrediting body for colleges and universities as a whole or for a specific program offered by such an institution. (Colleges and universities, incidentally, are evaluated and accredited overall—as a totality—by one of six regional or national accrediting associations, each of which is responsible for colleges and universities located in a particular geographical region of the United States—e.g., the Middle States Association of Colleges and Schools.)

Two groups that can recognize accrediting organizations or agencies as "reliable authorities as to the quality of training offered by educational institutions" (Standards for federal funding, 1972, p. 547) are the Council on Postsecondary Accreditation and the U.S. Commissioner of Education.

Both of these have recognized the American Speech-Language-Hearing Association as "the national accrediting agency for college and university programs offering *master's degrees* [italics mine] in speech pathology and audiology" (Standards for federal funding, 1972, p. 548). There were no organizations or agencies specifically accrediting baccalaurate or doctoral programs in these areas when this chapter was written.

Whether a college or university training program is accredited by an organization recognized by a national governmental unit can affect the flow of federal dollars to that program. Accreditation by such a body has sometimes been made a requirement for eligibility to participate in funding programs sponsored by agencies of the federal government, including those providing training grants (Oulahan, 1978). The Social and Rehabilitation Services Program of the Department of Health, Education, and Welfare during the early 1970s, for example, proposed to include the following in its list of criteria for determining eligibility for speech-language pathology and audiology training programs to participate in their training grants program:

> In order for master's degree programs to be eligible for support, they should be accredited, or be in the process of review for accreditation, by the American Speech and Hearing Association [now the American Speech-Language-Hearing Association] through the American Board of Examiners in Speech Pathology and Audiology and its Education and Training Board (Standards for Federal Funding, 1972, p. 546).

The use of such a criterion when determining eligibility of training programs for federal support has been questioned on the basis that it tends to create a *Catch 22* situation—that is, some unaccredited programs probably could be strengthened sufficiently with federal support to achieve accreditation, but their lack of accreditation impedes their securing the federal support they need to strengthen their curriculums. Such a situation was claimed to have existed during the early 1970s for some speech-language pathology and audiology training programs in predominantly black institutions (Standards for federal funding, 1972).

The functioning of both institutional and programmatic accrediting organizations is being subjected to increasing scrutiny. Their decisions are more frequently being viewed as judgments make by human beings (in most cases, human beings who are attempting to function in a relatively unbiased manner) rather than as facts or truths. Partial support for this conclusion can be found in the increasing amount of litigation in which accrediting organizations are defendants (Oulahan, 1978).

Further information of a general nature about accreditation can be found in the following papers: Oulahan (1978), Roemer (1974), and *Study of Accreditation of Selected Health Education Programs — Commission Report* (1973). For additional information about accreditation of speech-language pathology and audiology master's degree training programs, see Standards for accreditation of educational programs (1990).

Types of Regulation Administered by a Governmental Agency

There are three main ways by which a governmental agency can regulate the practice of an occupation: individual licensure, institutional licensure, and registration. The first was used most frequently to regulate the practice of speech-language pathology and audiology when this chapter was written.

Individual Licensure. Individual licensing laws are "a legal mechanism by which a governmental agency authorizes persons who have met specified minimal standards of competency to engage in a given profession or occupation" (Roemer, 1974, p. 26). Such laws can make licensure either mandatory or voluntary. If they are mandatory, they require all persons who practice the occupation or profession in the state to be licensed. If, on the other hand, they are voluntary, an unlicensed person can practice, but he or she cannot claim to be licensed. Voluntary licensure, therefore, can be viewed as a form of *governmental certification* (Roemer, 1974). Most state licensure laws that regulate the practice of speech-language pathology and audiology are of the mandatory type.

The standards under which an occupation is licensed in a particular state are specified in a statute enacted by the legislature in that state. This statute, among other things, establishes a new licensing board for that occupation or assigns it to an existing board. This board which functions as (or under the auspices of) an administrative agency, has the responsibility for implementing the licensure program mandated by the statute. Its members are unlikely to all be practitioners of the occupation. Consumers of its services are likely to be included. The board is almost always required by the state to be self-supporting, with expenses met by licensing fees. Such fees for a particular occupation can vary considerably from state to state. Their magnitude, in part, would be a function of the number of persons residing in the state who are likely to seek licensure for that occupation—the larger the number of such persons, the lower the fees are apt to be (Governmental regulation, 1969).

The formulation and passage of a state occupational licensing law (particularly one that is mandatory) is likely to cost the practitioners of the occupation (usually through their state association) a great deal, in terms of both time and money. They are likely to have to retain a lobbyist to guide their bill through the legislative process, and they have no guarantee that the lobbyist's efforts will be successful. If they are successful, practitioners will have to pay a license fee. Considering the financial and time investments involved, why would they seek to have their occupation licensed? Several possible reasons are suggested in the following paragraphs.

> The primary justification for licensure is the protection of the public. Protection of the public has broader implications than physical damage or loss of life. Unless it can be shown that the public needs protection, attempts to secure licensing regulations are not likely to succeed. . . .
> In addition to the primary justification mentioned above, there are other important reasons for desiring legislation. For example, licensure of a profession is perhaps the most stringent defense against encroachment on its activities by another profession . . . Further, licensing legislation tends to force rigorous definition of the activity involved. Finally, the economic advantages of licensure to the licensed group have been clearly recognized (Governmental regulation, 1969, p. 41).

The fact that the practitioners of an occupation have succeeded in having a state legislature pass a licensure law does not necessarily mean that their involvement with the that legislature has ended. They may have to ask it as some future time to change the requirements for licensure so that these requirements are consistent with how practitioners are being trained. (If the legislation itself is "vague," it may be possible for such changes to be made by the licensing board.) They may also have to convince it to not allow their licensure program to terminate. Some states have *sunset laws* under which entities such as occupational licensing boards are terminated at the end of a specified number of years unless the legislature acts to retain them (Survey of sunset laws, 1991). A legislature is unlikely to act to retain an agency unless it can be convinced that the agency is performing an essential function. Obviously, if an occupational licensing board is scheduled to be terminated and the practitioners of that occupation want it to be retained, they are going to have to convince the members of the legislature that it has been performing such a function. (For further information about sunset laws and occupational licensing, see Downey, 1979.)

A number of states have passed licensing laws or are seeking to pass licensing laws for speech-language pathologists and audiologists (see Heitman, 1980; Lynch, 1988, 1990; Lynch & Dubinske, 1986; Perspectives on licensure, 1986). Requirements for being licensed under these laws are summarized in Lynch (1990).

Institutional Licensure. Institutional licensure has existed for more than thirty-five years. Originally, it was concerned almost exclusively with the quality of facilities (e.g., sanitation and fire safety). Under this form of licensure certain aspects of the functioning of an institution (e.g., a nursing home, hospital, or rehabilitation center) are monitored by a government agency; so long as the institution conforms to certain minimum standards, it remains licensed to perform its function. The agency would tend to more concerned about whether its standards were being met than it would about the means by which they were being met. So long as the institution meets them by lawful means, the agency is unlikely to interfere.

There have been attempts since the early 1970s to extend institutional licensure to include regulating the quality of services provided by an institution (Levine, 1978). Although these attempts for the most part have been unsuccessful, they may foreshadow a movement that at some future time could affect the practice of speech-language pathology and audiology. Such a movement could have considerable impact on practitioners in these professions because the agency monitoring hospitals, rehabilitation centers, nursing homes, and other institutions providing clinical speech, language, and/or hearing services is likely to have its focus on the quality of the services provided—that is, whether they meet *minimum* standards with regard to quality. If the speech, language, and hearing services provided by an institution met the agency's minimum standards, it may not be concerned about whether the persons providing them are licensed in a particular manner by the state or certified by their professional association (particularly the latter). The institution, in a sense, would be responsible for establishing qualifications for persons providing the various services that it offers. Such qualifications may or may not conform to those for individual licensure or certification.

Institutional licensure, *if it were adopted*, could have a significant impact on the practice of speech-language pathology and audiology in medical settings. A hospital, for example, may hire a person who has a bachelor's degree with a major in speech-language pathology or audiology to do basic hearing testing. So long as the hospital could demonstrate that the person was capable of doing such hearing testing with results that possessed at least minimally acceptable levels of validity and reliability and that the person would refer cases requiring more sophisticated testing than he or she could provide, the government agency monitoring the institution would be unlikely to be concerned about the fact that the services were being provided by someone who was neither licensed nor certified in audiology. In fact, it is conceivable that the institution would be commended for not using an expensive, "overqualified" person to provide these services.

Most organizations representing health-related professionals are opposed to that aspect of institutional licensure concerned with establishing qualifications for personnel (Levine, 1978). They fear that some institutions, to reduce costs, might be tempted to hire practitioners who lack the qualifications for securing what they consider to be the appropriate state license or professional certification. They also have reservations about the ability of those doing the hiring at institutions (who may not be practitioners in their field) to establish qualifications for serving as practitioners in their field if they choose not to use the qualifications for the existing state license or professional certificate. Because of the less than enthusiastic reception that the concept of institutional licensure for personnel has received in many professional circles, it is doubtful that it will replace individual licensure or certification in the near future. It is likely, however, to *coexist* with them in a limited form. (This has already occurred at some institutions with regard to the paraprofessional designated as a *communication aid.* The qualifications for persons functioning in this role are established by the institutions employing them.)

Registration. Registration is a form of certification that is administered by a governmental agency. Persons who have completed the training deemed necessary by the agency to function as a practitioner in a particular field have their names listed in a register (file) that is maintained by that agency. A person may be able to become registered by graduating from a training program that is accredited by the agency.

The certificates that speech-language pathologists obtain from state departments of public instruction that allow them to work in public schools can be viewed as a form of registration. They may be registered almost automatically by completing a training program that is accredited by this state agency.

Registration has also been used in another way for regulating the practice of speech-language pathology and audiology. Some states (e.g., Wisconsin) have used it as a first step to licensing them after passage of a licensure law.

WHAT APPROACHES HAVE BEEN USED TO REGULATE THE PRACTICE OF SPEECH-LANGUAGE PATHOLOGY AND AUDIOLOGY?

This far in this chapter we have explored both the motivation for regulating the practice of an occupation and the approaches that have been used for this purpose. This section deals with the manner in which these approaches have been used for regulating the practice of speech-language pathology and audiology. The information presented in quite general because the requirements for certification, licensure, accreditation, and registration in these fields have been and are likely to continue to be revised frequently.

Certification

The professional association that is most actively involved in the clinical certification of speech-language pathologists and audiologists is the American Speech-Language-Hearing Association (ASHA). ASHA has been certifying the clinical competence of practitioners in communicative disorders since the early 1950s. It currently offers two Certificates of Clinical Competence—one in speech-language pathology and one in audiology. Both require an applicant to have earned a master's degree, to have completed a prescribed program of academic and practicum experience in a graduate program accredited by ASHA, to have completed a clinical fellowship year (i.e., an internship), to have agreed to conform to a code of ethics, and to have passed a national examination (Implementation procedures for the standards for the Certificates of Clinical Competence, 1991). Write to the American Speech-Language-Hearing Association for specific information concerning the requirements for these certificates.

While ASHA did not offer *specialty certification* when this chapter was written, it did have an *ad hoc* committee looking into the need for it (Kenneth Moll, personal communication). Several groups of interest to speech-language pathologists and audiologists have offered specialty certification for the administration and interpretation of a diagnostic test—e.g., the *Porch Test of Communicative Ability* (Porch, 1967).

Accreditation

The American Speech-Language-Hearing Association maintains an accreditation program for master's degree training programs in speech-language pathology and audiology (Standards for accreditation of educational programs, 1990). Both a listing of accredited programs and specific information about requirements for accreditation can be obtained from ASHA. The American Speech-Language-Hearing also maintains an accreditation program for professional services programs (see Council on professional standards, 1991).

Licensure

A number of states require speech-language pathologists and audiologists to be licensed (see Lynch, 1990) and have established agencies (boards) for this purpose. [Members of state licensure boards for our field coordinate their activities through the National Council of State Boards of Examiners for Speech-Language Pathology and Audiology— see Norman, 1986.] The specific requirements for licensure (if a state requires it) can be obtained from the state board responsible for administering the program. Information about state licensure for speech-language pathologists and audiologists is published in the *Asha* journal, the *Governmental Affairs Review* (published by ASHA), and in the *Licensure Newsletter*, which is published by The National Council of State Boards of Examiners for Speech-Language Pathology and Audiology (P.O. Box 326, Wellsburg, WV 26070). For an historical review of the development of licensure for our field, see Cooper (1991).

Registration

The certification that a speech-language pathologist must obtain to be employable in the public schools of a particular state can be viewed as a form of registration. (The rationale for viewing it in this manner is presented elsewhere in this chapter.) The requirements for such certification vary widely from state to state. Those for a particular state can be obtained from its department of public instruction.

As mentioned earlier, several states (e.g., Wisconsin) have used registration to regulate the practice of speech-language pathology and audiology for a few years following the passage of a licensing law while the licensing board is being set up and specific requirements for licensure are being established.

HOW CAN CERTIFICATION, ACCREDITATION, LICENSURE, AND REGISTRATION BE LOST?

When individuals have achieved certification, licensure, or registration or when training programs have been accredited, it is tempting for them to assume that their new status is permanent. This is not necessarily true! Certification, licensure, registration, and accreditation can be lost for a variety of reasons. Some of the more common ones are described in this section.

Reasons for Loss of Certification, Licensure, and Registration

Failure to Abide by the Code of Ethics. A requirement for any form of occupational certification, licensure, or registration is agreeing to be ethical in one's interactions with consumers and follow professionals. Unfortunately, the categorization of behavior as ethical or unethical involves a value judgment—there probably is no behavior that would be categorized as either ethical or unethical by most persons under all circumstances. This being the case, how does a governmental agency or a professional association determine whether particular behavior is unethical? They usually do this by operationally defining (Bridgman, 1961) behaving ethically as adhering to a code of ethics. The code of ethics describes a set of behaviors that can occur in interactions between practitioners and consumers and between practitioners and other professionals, some of which are to be regarded as ethical and others as unethical. If a practitioner does something that is *prohibited* by the code of ethics or fails to do something that the code of ethics *requires*, the practitioner can be classified as behaving in an unethical manner and can lose his or her license, certification, or registration. This appears to be one of the main reasons why persons lose their ASHA certification (see Actions of the ethical practice board, 1986, 1988, 1989a, 1989b, 1991). For further information about codes of professional ethics see Chapter 3.

Failure to Maintain Membership in the Certifying Organization or to Pay Required Fees. Some certifying organizations (including the American Speech-Language-Hearing Association) require persons to whom they award certification to either maintain membership in them or to pay an annual fee, which is regarded as their fair share of the costs to the organization of maintaining the certification program. Failure to do so can result in loss of certification. Similarly, failure to pay licensing and registration fees (if there are any) can result in loss of these credentials.

Failure to Comply with Changes in Requirements for the Certification, Licensure, or Registration. The requirements for a given type of certification, licensure, or registration are likely to change from time to time. Are persons who are already certified, licensed, or registered required to meet new requirements? The answer to this question depends on whether there is a *grandfather clause* and, if there is, what it covers. A grandfather clause excuses a person who is already certified, licensed, or registered from having to meet some new requirements, but not necessarily all new requirements. Such a clause, for example, would be unlikely to excuse one from a new requirement for participation in continuing education.

The Certification, Licensure, or Registration Being Terminated. A person may lose one of these credentials because the program under which it was awarded is terminated. Of the three, a speech-language pathologist or audiologist is most likely to lose licensure in this manner. A number of states have enacted sunset laws (Downey, 1979) that affect their licensure boards. When there is such a law, a licensure board is automatically terminated after a certain number of years unless the legislature votes to continue it.

Reasons for Loss of Accreditation

A training program can lose its accreditation for several reasons, singly or in combination. First, it can be judged to no longer be meeting the standards under which it was accredited. This can happen if faculty leave and are not replaced by persons who, in the judgment of the accrediting agency, are competent to teach their courses. Second, the program can be judged as unable to meet some of the standards which are new that are in effect when it is considered for reaccreditation. The accreditation awarded by most organizations, including the American Speech-Language-Hearing Association, is for a finite number of years. If a training program wishes to remain accredited, it must apply for reaccreditation at the end of this period. And third, it may not apply for reaccreditation when its accreditation terminates because, for example, the faculty do not believe that it meets current standards for accreditation. The program, of course, can attempt to meet these standards at a later date and reapply.

PROCEDURES USED FOR TAKING AWAY ACCREDITATION, LICENSURE, AND REGISTRATION

The procedures that are used by a professional association or governmental agency for taking away the license, registration, or certification of a practitioner or the accreditation of a training program are supposed to be consistent with the concept of *due process* (specifically, procedural due process) which can be viewed as one of the cornerstones of our legal system (Morris, 1984). If due process is being adhered to in such procedures, the person or training program in question will be informed of the charges that have been made and will be given an opportunity to answer them. This can involve a hearing during which the agency or association and the individual or training program present evidence to a hearing officer supporting their contentions that the credential should and should not be taken away. Both parties are likely to be represented by attorneys. Following presentation of the evidence, the hearing officer (who is supposed to be unbiased) decides whether the *preponderance of evidence* supports the charges made by the agency or association. If in his or her judgment the preponderance of evidence supports the charges that were made, the hearing officer can order the licensure, registration, certification, or accreditation be taken away. Of course, a hearing officer probably would not order revocation if he or she felt that the charges, though proven, were not serious enough to warrant such action.

If the person or training program involved feels that the decision of the hearing officer was not warranted by the evidence which was presented, the person or program has the right to appeal it. At least one level of appeal is usually possible within the agency or association. If the person or training program remains dissatisfied after exhausting all internal possibilities for appeal, a civil suit against the agency or association can be initiated in an appropriate state or federal court. The procedures by which this would be done are outlined in Chapter 2.

In some cases the charges made can be answered without the need for a formal hearing. The association or agency can present the person or program with a written statement of the charges and ask that he, she, or the program *show cause* (in writing) why the credential should not be taken away. If it is obvious that the charges lack merit, it should be possible to resolve the situation in this manner. The American Speech-Language-Hearing Association has used this approach in its clinical certification and accreditation programs.

Write to the American Speech-Language-Hearing Association for specific information about appeals procedures in its clinical certification and accreditation programs. For comparable information about state licensure and registration programs, contact the appropriate agency (licensing board or department of public instruction).

Chapter V

CONTRACTUAL OBLIGATIONS TO CLIENTS AND OTHERS

In our society it is almost impossible to be completely self-sufficient. We rely on others to provide almost all of the goods and services we consume. This mandatory reliance on others has several implications. First, it means we need a mechanism to ensure that a person who agrees to provide us with certain goods and services does what he or she promises. And second, it means we need a mechanism for ensuring that a person who provides goods and services for another will be fairly compensated for them (usually by being given money). The legal mechanism used in our society to enforce promises is the *contract*. Without a mechanism for enforcing promises, a society such as ours in which we must rely on others to satisfy most of our needs would be impossible.

We are constantly entering into contracts in both our personal and professional lives. We often are not consciously aware of doing so because we tend to view contracts as written documents that must be signed to be enforceable. A contract *does not* have to be written to be enforceable. Under certain circumstances *oral promises* (both direct and implied) and those that are indicated by out nonverbal behavior are enforceable as contracts. Also, some written documents that are labeled contracts are *not enforceable*. Thus, some promises that appear to be enforceable as contracts are not and others that do not appear to be enforceable as contracts are enforceable as contracts. Since we cannot avoid entering into contracts, we must be able to recognize when we are doing so and what the implications are. My overall objective in this chapter is to increase your level of awareness and understanding of the contracts you enter into, particularly those you enter into while functioning as a speech-language pathologist or audiologist.

EVENTS THAT CAN RESULT IN
THE CREATION OF A CONTRACT

A contract is an *enforceable promise*. It is described in the authoritative work, *Restatement of the Law: Contracts,* in the following manner: "A contract is a promise for the breach of which the law gives a remedy, or the performance of which the law in some way recognizes as a duty" (1973, p. 5). Thus, a contract is a promise (or a set of promises) that a court is likely to enforce if it is asked to do so. The qualifier "is likely" was used here because the courts do not always do what they would be expected to do. Also, the phrase "if it is asked to do so" was added because a court cannot become involved in the enforcement of a contract unless the person to whom the promise that was not kept was made initiates a civil suit (see Chapter 2 for a discussion of civil suits). The threat of such a suit, incidentally, may be enough to motivate a person to do what he or she promised, for being a defendant in a suit that is likely to be successful can be expensive (because of attorney's fees and court costs).

Contracts also have been defined as *enforceable agreements.* When people enter into a contractual relationship they usually agree to do certain things for each other. For example, an audiologist agrees to test a child's hearing, and the parents agree to pay him or her a certain amount of money for performing this service. The word "agreement" sometimes is used in written contracts instead of the word "contract."

What role does contract law play in our legal system? As we saw in Chapter 2 the laws that make up our legal system impose *restrictions and obligations* on our behavior. These restrictions and obligations are of two types: involuntary and voluntary. We are required to behave in a manner consistent with the first type, which are the majority, *regardless of whether we have promised or agreed to do so.* (We indirectly promise or agree to do so by residing in our country and thereby in our state and municipality.) The sources of such laws (restrictions and obligations) include federal, state, and municipal legislatures, administrative agencies, and court decisions (i.e., common law).

The second type of law that imposes restrictions and obligations on our behavior we voluntarily agree to obey. These laws are created by *private individuals* rather than legislatures or government agencies. They are private rather than public laws. They can impose restrictions and obligations on the behavior of only a relative small number of persons—

often as few as two. They do not duplicate public laws but supplement them. Thus, contract law provides a mechanism for imposing restrictions and obligations on behavior in some situations—interactions between people—that are not regulated by public law.

Though contracts are private laws, they are enforced by the courts, the same institution that enforces public laws. The courts have established rules for *creating and enforcing* contracts. A contract that is created in a manner consistent with these rules is highly likely to be enforced by the courts. Hence, it is necessary to understand these rules in order to understand how certain events can result in the creation of a contract. My objective in this section is to help you to develop an intuitive understanding of some of the more important of these rules, particularly those pertaining to the *three events* that are necessary for creating a contract: (1) the *offer*, or promise, (2) the *acceptance* of the offer, and (3) the exchange of *consideration* by the parties—i.e., the voluntarily relinquishing of something by each party (e.g., time or money).

The Offer (Promise)

The first event that occurs for a contract to be created is the act of *making an offer*. A speech-language pathologist, for example, can offer to include an adult stutterer in an ongoing group therapy program. The person who makes the offer is referred to as the *offeror* and the person to whom it is made is referred to as the *offeree*. Thus, the speech-language pathologist in this example would be the offeror and the adult stutterer would be the offeree.

The offer-making process almost always involves the offeror conveying to the offeree (1) what he or she will do for the offeree and (2) what he or she expects in return from the offeree. The word "conveying" was used here rather than "saying" and/or "writing" because an offer can be communicated without the use of spoken or written language. It can be conveyed by implication. Thus, "A promise may be stated in words either oral or written, or may be inferred wholly or partially from conduct" (*Restatement of the Law: Contracts*, 1973, p. 12). The following is an example of a situation in which an offer is conveyed without words:

> A [letter designates a person], on passing a market, where he has an account, sees a box of apples marked "5 cts. each." A picks up an apple, holds it up so that a clerk of the establishment sees the act. The clerk nods, and A passes on. A has promised to pay five cents for the apple (*Restatement of the Law: Contracts*, 1973, pp. 12–13).

Similarly, a hard-of-hearing adult who seeks and accepts a hearing aid evaluation from an audiologist conveys to that audiologist by implication a promise to pay him or her (or have a third party do so) a reasonable fee for the evaluation. The presumption in our society is that people are willing to pay a reasonable fee for professional services they ask for and receive.

Theoretically, it should be a relatively easy task to determine whether an offer has been made. All one should have to establish is whether a promise was conveyed from offeror to offeree by words, or by implication, or by some combination of the two. Unfortunately, this may not be an easy task. It depends on what an objective observer (i.e., "reasonable person") would have perceived to be the *intent* of the offeror when he or she said, or wrote, or did what could be construed as an offer. According to Fisher:

> Whether an offer has been made depends on *intent* — the objective intent of a reasonable man observing the actions claimed to constitute the offer. It is not the subjective intent of the offeror that controls the determination of whether an offer has been made (1977, p. 418).

Thus, when attempting to determine whether an offer has been made a judge would consider if a *reasonable person* hearing or seeing the words or observing the actions that are claimed to have conveyed the offer would conclude that an offer had been made. If the judge feels that a *reasonable person* would have been likely to perceive those words and/or actions as conveying an offer, he or she probably will rule that the intent was to make an offer. On the other hand, if the judge feels that a *reasonable person* would have been unlikely to perceive those words and/or actions as conveying an offer, he or she probably will rule that they do not constitute an offer. Since there probably will be no way for the judge to establish the *subjective* intent of the offeror, the judge, one would hope, will not include what he or she thinks the intent was as a factor in the decision (i.e., ruling).

It is desirable that offers be as specific, or unambiguous, as possible. The more specific an offer, the more likely both offeror and offeree will agree on what is being proposed, that is, the obligations they will be expected to assume if the offer is accepted. Also, if an offer is accepted and becomes a contract, a court will have less difficulty determining whether the contract has been breached (violated) if the language is relatively specific, or unambiguous. In this regard, it is particularly important that when a speech-language pathologist or audiologist offers clinical services to a communicatively handicapped person, the person and/or the family understands that the offer does not promise (guarantee) a cure or a specific level of improvement. All that can be promised (guaranteed) is that the speech-language pathologist or audiologist will make a reasonable attempt to assist the person in reducing the severity of the communicative disorder for as long a period as it is reasonable to expect significant improvement to be possible. A judge would be unlikely to view the failure of speech-language pathology or audiology services to significantly reduce the severity of a person's communicative disorder to constitute a *breach of contract* if a reasonable attempt was made to assist the person in reducing its severity. However, a judge would be likely to view this as a breach of contract if clinical services were being provided when there was little hope for significant improvement (unless the person or family, after being informed that the prognosis for further improvement was extremely poor, requested *in writing* that therapy services be continued). Providing a client with clinical services when there is no reasonable hope for improvement could also be viewed as a violation of the American Speech-Language-Hearing Association's Code of Ethics (see Chapter 3).

An offer must be *formally communicated* before it can be accepted and lead to the formation of a contract. What constitutes formal communication is the use of a medium (such as a letter) that is normally used for communicating such offers. If you heard "through the grapevine" that you had been awarded a grant for which you had applied, you ordinarily could not sue those awarding it for breach of contract if they changed their mind before formally communicating (probably in writing) to you an offer of the award.

An offeror usually can withdraw, or terminate, an offer during the period between when it is communicated to the offeree and the offeree formally accepts it. There are a variety of reasons an offeror might do this. One is particularly relevant to clinical practice—that is, *lapse of a reasonable time.* A person who is offered clinical services by a speech-language pathologist or audiologist should be given a reasonable period of time to decide whether to accept them. When the services are offered, the prospective client should be told how much time he or she has to accept the offer. If the client does not accept within this time period, the clinician is no longer obliged to either reserve a slot in the schedule for the person or to provide the services offered for the agreed fee.

Acceptance of the Offer

The second event that must occur for a contract to be formed is the *acceptance* of the offer by the offeree. An adult stutterer, for example, may accept a speech-language pathologist's offer to enroll him or her in a therapy group.

If an offeree wishes to accept an offer and thereby establish a contract, how should he or she do it? "Acceptance of an offer is a manifestation of assent to the terms thereof made by the offeree in a manner invited or required by the offer" (*Restatement of the Law: Contracts*, 1973, p. 108). Thus, an offeree can accept an offer—that is, the *totality* of what has been offered—by indicating a desire to do so in the manner specified by the offeror (e.g., by signing a contract). If the offeror does not specify how acceptance should be manifested, then any reasonable mode can be used.

There are two basic ways by which acceptance of an offer can be manifested, or indicated. The first of these is acceptance by *performance*. "Acceptance by performance requires that at least part of what the offer requests be performed or tendered" (*Restatement of the Law: Contracts*, 1973, p. 108). Thus, an offeree can indicate acceptance *without words* by beginning to do what acceptance of the offer would require him or her to do, assuming the offer has not been withdrawn or terminated. An adult stutterer could accept a speech-language pathologist's offer of enrollment in a particular ongoing therapy group by attending one or more sessions of that group. Or an audiologist could accept an offer to screen the hearing of the children enrolled in a private school by beginning to screen their hearing.

The second way acceptance can be manifested is by a *promise*. "Acceptance by a promise requires that the offeree complete every act essential to the making of the promise" (*Restatement of the Law: Contracts*, 1973, p. 108). In this case, an offeree would accept an offer by *promising* to do what is required by the offer. He or she may make the promise in words or other symbols (e.g., manual signs) or may imply the promise by conduct. A speech-language pathologist or audiologist in private practice would be accepting an offer by making a promise when he or she signed a *lease* for an office (the lease being a contract). The promise would include the payment of a certain amount of money to the offeror for rent each month for the duration of the lease.

The courts ordinarily do not interpret an offeree's *silence* (i.e., failure to notify the offeror that he or she does not want to accept the offer) as conveying acceptance. Thus, if a speech-language pathologist told an adult stutterer that she will assume the stutterer wants to be enrolled in the therapy group unless she is informed to the contrary before the end of the month, she would be on shaky ground. The courts usually will rule that an offer has not been accepted unless the offeree conveys acceptance by performance or by making a promise. One of the few exceptions that speech-language pathologists and audiologists are likely to encounter pertains to delivery of the "main selection" in book clubs. Many of these clubs will send you the main selection *offered* each month if you *fail to notify* them within a specified period of time that you don't want it. Here silence after being offered the main selection is interpreted as indicating acceptance of the offer because you agreed to it being interpreted in this manner when you joined.

The offeree must accept the offer in its *entirety* for a contract to be formed. If an offeree is willing to accept parts of it, he or she can convey to the offeror a statement of the parts that he or she is willing to accept. This statement would be regarded as a *counteroffer*. The making of a counteroffer terminates the offeror's original offer.

The Consideration Exchanged by the Parties

Acceptance of an offer will only result in the formation of a contract *if certain conditions are met*. (An in-depth discussion of these conditions is presented in the volumes *Corbin on Contracts*, 1952, and *Restatement of the Law: Contracts*, 1973.) One of the most important is that *consideration* be exchanged by the parties. "Consideration embraces the idea that there should be a voluntary relinquishment of a known right by the respective parties to one another for there to be an enforceable agreement by either of them against the other" (Fisher, 1977, p. 449). The courts tend to view it as only fair that *both* offeror and offeree voluntarily agree to give up something (i.e., to assume an obligation that would not have to be assumed if there were no contract). The courts ordinarily will not enforce a contract in which one or both parties failed to voluntarily relinquish a known right.

What constitutes consideration perhaps can be made clearer by describing the two forms it can take. The first is that the offeree agrees to give up something that belongs to the offeree that could *benefit the offeror*. For example, a hard-of-hearing person (offeror) offers to buy a hearing aid from an audiologist (offeree) for $500. The audiologist accepts the offer and delivers the hearing aid. The transfer and delivery of the hearing aid constitutes consideration because in exchange for a promise to pay $500 the audiologist has voluntarily relinquished something that he owns (a hearing aid) that should benefit the hard-of-hearing person. The hard-of-hearing person, in turn, would be voluntarily relinquishing something that belongs to him — $500.

The *second form* that consideration can take is that the offeree in accepting an offer agrees to do something that would be recognized by the courts as having a *detrimental* effect on him or her (i.e., cause the offeree to do something he or she wouldn't choose to do) rather than having a beneficial effect on the offeror. The following example illustrates this form of consideration:

> A promises B, his nephew aged 16, that A will pay B $1000 when B becomes 21 if B does not smoke before then. B's forebearance to smoke is a performance and if bargained for is consideration for A's promise (*Restatement of the Law: Contracts*, 1973, p. 152).

The phrase *bargained for,* as used here, implies that the money offered was not merely a gift. The assumption is being made that B would have smoked if his uncle hadn't made the offer. Thus, in not smoking he would voluntarily be relinquishing a right. It, of course, could be argued that the uncle was receiving a psychological benefit — that is, not having to cope with a nephew who smokes.

For an act to constitute consideration, what is being relinquished by performing the act must be an *actual* (real) known right. Agreeing to do for someone something that one is required to do by law ordinarily would not constitute consideration. Since we are expected to meet our legal obligations, then doing something we are obliged to do anyway would not constitute relinquishing a known right. Thus, in the following example there is no act that is likely to be construed by a court as constituting consideration since a police officer has a legal duty to produce evidence.

> A offers a reward to whoever produces evidence leading to the arrest and conviction of the murderer of B. C produces such evidence in the performance of his duty as a police officer. C's performance is not consideration for A's promise (*Restatement of the Law: Contracts*, 1973, p. 157).

If a public school speech-language pathologist made an offer to the parents of a language-handicapped child to include their child in her caseload in exchange for an hourly fee and they accepted, she probably would be unsuccessful in suing the parents for breach of contract if they refused to pay her the money after she did so. The clinician was not relinquishing a right by offering to provide clinical services for the child because her contract with the school district required her to do so.

Events That Can Interfere with the Creation of an Enforceable Contract

There are several reasons, other than a problem with consideration, that can lead to the acceptance of an offer not resulting in an enforceable contract. They will be dealt with briefly in this section. For additional information about them see Corbin (1952), Fisher (1977), and *Restatement of the Law: Contracts* (1973).

The reasons referred to in the preceding paragraph include the following: (1) incapacity, (2) fraud, (3) mistake, (4) duress, (5) the offer being unconscionable, (6) illegality, and (7) the contract not being in written form when it was required to be. A court may legally excuse a party to a contract from meeting his or her contractual obligations if it can be established that *there is no contract* because of one or more of these reasons. For the acceptance of an offer to result in the creation of a contract *the assumption has to be made* that the parties have the mental and legal *capacity* to enter into a contract, that one party is not attempting to commit a *fraud* on the other, that the offer actually was accepted and the contract reflects the agreement (i.e., it contains no *mistakes* that can influence its interpretation), that the offeree did not accept the offer under *duress,* and so forth. A court is likely to rule that no contract exists and, hence, neither party can seek damages for it being breached if the *preponderance of evidence* suggests that this assumption is not viable. These reasons why acceptance of an offer may not result in an enforceable contract are of more than academic interest. They can provide you with a legal means to escape from the obligations a contract calls for you to assume. They also can cause a court to nullify a contract in which you are the offeror.

Incapacity. The law requires that a person who is accepting an offer have the *mental capacity* to understand the obligations he or she is assuming for the acceptance to result in the formation of a contract. If it can be established that a person lacks such mental capacity, a court is likely to rule that any contracts he or she enters into are unenforceable.

Several categories of persons are almost always assumed by the courts to lack the mental capacity needed to knowledgeably enter into at least some contractual relationships. These include persons who have not yet reached the *age of majority* (children) and persons who are intoxicated.

Also included are persons who have been diagnosed as *mentally ill* or *mentally defective.*

A person usually can escape from having to meet at least some contractual obligations by reason of mental incapacity if one or both of the following can be established:

(a) he is unable to understand in a reasonable manner the nature and consequences of the transaction, or

(b) he is unable to act in a reasonable manner in relation to the transaction and the other party has reason to know of his condition (*Restatement of the Law: Contracts,* 1973, p. 33).

One or both probably could be established for persons diagnosed as moderately or severely mentally retarded or for those diagnosed as senile. It may also be possible to establish one or both for persons who have certain communicative disorders resulting from damage to the central nervous system. It could be argued, for example, that a severe receptive aphasic who accepted an offer was "unable to understand in a reasonable manner the nature and consequences of the transaction." A speech-language pathologist, incidentally, might be asked to testify whether in his or her professional opinion it is likely that a particular receptive aphasic who entered into a contract was able to do so. (See Chapter 11 for a discussion of the role of the speech-language pathologist or audiologist as an *expert witness.*)

Mental capacity, as defined by these two criteria, is also of concern to audiologists. It could be argued, for example, that a deaf person who does not speechread well and accepted an oral offer was "unable to understand in a reasonable manner the nature and consequences of the transaction." For an in-depth discussion of the implications of the offeree being deaf on the acceptance of an offer (and, hence, on the creation of a contract), see Section 12 in Meyers' (1968) book, *The Law and the Deaf.*

The courts may be unwilling to allow someone to escape from meeting all contractual obligations because of mental incapacity. They may rule that a person is mentally competent to enter into some contractual relationships but not into others. Also, a person may be unable to avoid meeting contractual obligations because the offeror was unaware of his or her mental condition. Some of the issues involved in determining competency are summarized in the following paragraph from the authoritative work, *Restatement of the Law: Contracts:*

The *standard of competency*. It is now recognized that there is a wide variety of types and degrees of mental incompetency. Among them are congenital deficiencies in intelligence, the mental deterioration of old age, *the effects of brain damage caused by accident or organic disease* [italics mine], and mental illness evidenced by such symptoms as delusions, hallucinations, delirium, confusion, and depression. Where no guardian has been appointed [by a court], there is full contractual capacity in any case unless the mental disease or defect has affected the particular transaction: a person may be able to understand almost nothing, or only simple or routine transactions, or he may be incompetent only with respect to a particular type of transaction. Even though understanding is complete, he may lack capacity to control his acts in the way that the normal individual can and does control them; in such cases the incapacity makes the contract voidable only if the other party has reason to know of his condition. Where a person has some understanding of a particular transaction which is affected by mental illness or defect, the controlling consideration is whether the transaction in its result is one which a reasonably competent person might have made (1973, p. 34).

Fraud. Fraud is "an intentional perversion of truth for the purpose of inducing another in reliance upon it to part with some valuable thing belonging to him or to surrender a legal right . . . " (Black, 1968, p. 788). An offeror committing a fraud would *intentionally* provide false information to the offeree to induce acceptance of an offer. The offeror by behaving in this manner is attempting to *defraud* the offeree.

A person who has been defrauded has several options. He or she can ask a court for a release from the contractual obligations—that is, ask the court to rule that no contract exists. Or the person can force the offeror to live up to the contractual obligations if he or she feels that this would be advantageous to him or her (or disadvantageous to the offeror). A contractual relationship that a person was induced to enter because of fraud may become one from which he or she can derive some benefit *because of a change in circumstances*. Suppose, for example, an audiologist agrees to screen the employees of a factory at some future time for $5000 after the company *intentionally* leads her to believe that the factory employs fewer people than it does. She finds out about this after signing the contract. When the time comes for her to do the screening, she is told that many of the employees have been laid off. Thus, because of a change in circumstances (i.e., fewer employees to screen) the fee she was promised would be more than adequate to compensate her for doing the screening. A court would be unlikely to release the company from its contractual obligation if asked to do so because it originally intended to defraud the audiologist. A judge, in fact, is apt to view enforcement of the contract as yielding poetic justice!

Mistake. A mistake is an *"unintentional* [italics mine] act, omission, or error arising from ignorance, surprise, . . . or misplaced confidence" (Black, 1968, p. 1152). A mistake made by either the offeror or offeree can result in a contract that one or both parties view as unfair.

Our concern here pertains to the impact "of action that has been induced by a mistaken thought" (Corbin, 1952, p. 539) on the enforceability of contracts. An offeree may accept an offer ("action") because he or she misunderstood (was mistaken about) what was being offered. Or the offeror may act on the belief that the offeree has accepted the offer when the offeree did not intend to do so. The offeror's action in such an instance would have been "induced by a mistaken thought." (This type of mistake, incidentally, can be prevented by having a written contract: The offeree by signing the contract indicates unequivocally that he or she wants to accept the offer.) Or a person may make an offer *in jest* that is accepted on the mistaken belief that it is a serious offer. Or an offeree may accept an offer (e.g., sign a contract) on the mistaken belief that the information presented in it is accurate, but the offeror *unintentionally* included inaccurate information in it. In all of these situations there is a *possibility* a court would rule that no contract exists because acceptance of the offer did not involve a true "meeting of minds." However, there is no guarantee that a court would rule there is no contract. There are circumstances under which a court is likely to rule that a contract is enforceable regardless of the fact that mistakes were made by the offeror, offeree, or both. An attorney should be able to advise you about whether you are likely to be successful in escaping from a contractual relationship that you entered because of a mistake.

While a court may release you from fulfilling a contract that did not involve a true "meeting of minds," it is unlikely to release you from fulfilling one you accepted but later found to be *disadvantageous*. The courts expect people to study offers carefully before accepting them (e.g., before signing contracts). While your not having done so may have been a *mistake*, a court is unlikely to declare a contract unenforceable for this reason.

Duress. The acceptance of an offer is supposed to be a *voluntary* act. A person is supposed to accept an offer because he or she rightly or wrongly views it as advantageous to do so. If a person accepts an offer because he or she actually or figuratively has "a gun held to his head," the courts are likely to rule that the offer was accepted under duress and, hence, the contract is void *unless the offeree wishes it to be enforced.* A person who forces someone to accept an offer may end up outsmarted because the contract may unexpectedly prove to be highly advantageous to the offeree. The offeree can insist on enforcement of the contract in such a case and sue the offeror for breach of contract if he or she fails to do what was promised. Such a situation would be one in which poetic justice prevailed.

The Offer is Unconscionable. Occasionally, a contract contains a clause (or clauses) that is so *unreasonably favorable* to the interests of one of the parties that a judge is likely to rule that the clause is unenforceable as it stands. A judge would be unlikely to rule part of a contract unconscionable unless it unequivocally violated his or her sense of fairness (see the discussion of natural law in Chapter 2). Being unconscionable is something beyond one party's bargaining more successfully and as a result getting a better deal. Judges usually are unwilling to rule parts clauses of contracts unconscionable unless the evidence is overwhelming.

Why would a person accept an offer that has aspects which are unconscionable? The only reason probably would be that he or she had no choice. A person who has a desperate need to borrow money but cannot borrow it from a bank because of a poor credit rating may be forced to borrow it from a loan shark at an extremely high interest rate. In the unlikely event that the loan shark sued the person for breach of contract for failure to pay the exorbitant interest rate agreed to, the judge would be likely to rule that the interest rate was unconscionable and, hence, the contract was unenforceable in its present form. To make it enforceable, the judge probably would order the interest rate reduced to one that he felt was fair.

Illegality. The courts will not enforce a contract that violates either criminal or civil law—that is, one that would result in the commission of a crime or a tort. (See Chapter 6 for a discussion of torts.)

The Contract is Not in Written Form. While it certainly is desirable for contracts to be written, for some types it is *essential.* The courts will not enforce them unless they are written. Included here are contracts for the sale of goods over a certain price and those that take longer than a certain period of time to complete. The amounts for both vary from state to state.

Possible Remedies for a Contract That is Breached

What options do you have if a person with whom you have a contract refuses to do what he or she promised? There are two possible strategies. The first would be to seek an *out-of-court settlement* and the second would be to sue for *breach of contract*. Most wronged parties initially would seek an out-of-court settlement: if this were not attainable, they would consider suing for breach of contract. The legal fees for out-of-court settlements tend to be less than for in-court suits.

The wronged party's objective, regardless of whether he or she is seeking an out-of-court or an in-court settlement, is *to attain the position he or she would have been in if the contract had been completed.* The most direct way that the wronged party can be put in this position is for the party who breached the contract to do voluntarily what was promised because he or she considers the cost of not doing to be too high. The term "cost" here refers not only to time and money, but also to such intangibles as *damage to one's reputation.* Other ways that a wronged party can be put in this position are by having the breaching party return what was received as *consideration* (i.e., by having him or her make *restitution*) or pay *compensatory damages* to offset the losses sustained by the contract not being completed.

Out-Of-Court Settlements. Before initiating a suit the wronged party will probably attempt to motivate the breaching party to do as promised, or return whatever was given as payment for doing what was promised, or to pay an amount of money that would compensate for any losses the wronged party sustained. To achieve this objective he or she may employ such motivational devices as a *letter from an attorney* which makes a direct or indirect threat to sue if the matter cannot be settled out of court. He or she may also threaten to *file a complaint* with an organization such as the *Better Business Bureau* if the matter is not resolved in a satisfactory manner or contact the consumer advocate at a local television station. One or more of these is often adequate to motivate the breaching party to behave in an equitable manner.

Suits for Breach of Contract. A suit for breach of contract is a civil suit and is conducted in the same manner as any other civil suit. The procedures by which such suits are initiated and conducted are described in Chapter 2. The plaintiff (the wronged party) may seek any of a number of *remedies* from the courts. The one that plaintiff's seek most often in breach of contract suits is *compensatory damages.* This consists of an award of money (from the defendant) that is intended to put the plaintiff in the financial position he or she would have been in if the contract had been completed.

CONTRACTUAL ASPECTS OF THE CLIENT–CLINICIAN RELATIONSHIP

The client-clinician relationship is, among other things, a contractual relationship. The offeror is the clinician and the offeree is the client or his or her family. (Throughout this discussion the term "client" will be assumed to include the client's family where relevant.) The consideration offered by the clinician usually is time and expertise. It could also be a device such as a hearing aid. That offered by the client is a promise to pay a fee for services rendered. The client may or may not be aware of the amount of this fee when treatment is begun. In some cases the fee is paid (partially or fully) by a third party such as a public school system or a medical insurance program (e.g., Medicare). The clinician *offers* a service to the client which the client *accepts*. The client is likely to conclude that the clinician has not breached the contract if the client receives from the clinician what he or she *thought* the clinician promised.

The problem most frequently encountered is probably that the client and the clinician have *different interpretations* of the offer. The client when accepting the offer interprets it to be what he or she *wants* it to be rather than what the clinician *intends* it to be. The offeror and offeree do not have a true "meeting of minds." Aside from the legal implications of this situation, it can adversely affect the therapy process.

One way that clients can misconstrue a clinician's offer is to interpret it as guaranteeing significant improvement. They may assume that the clinician by offering his or her services is *implicitly* promising that therapy will be helpful. The clinician, of course, cannot make such a promise for any of several reasons, including the fact that it would violate the ASHA Code of Ethics (see Chapter 3). It is crucial, therefore, that both the client and his or her family understand *before* therapy is initiated that improvement cannot be guaranteed. However, they should be given some estimate of the likelihood that it will be helpful.

Another way that a client and/or his or her family can misconstrue a clinician's offer is by assuming that the responsibility for the client's improving rests completely, or almost completely, on the clinician. They may expect the clinician to do things to the client that will cause the client to change in the manner they desire. Considering the nature of the therapy process, such an assumption is not realistic. Speech-language pathologists and audiologists almost always attempt to help their clients help themselves. The client is expected to assume an active rather than a passive role. It is crucial, therefore, that when therapy is offered, the client and the family be informed as specifically as possible about what the client would be expected to do. Clients should be told that if they are unable or unwilling to do what they are asked to by the clinician, they will probably be wasting their time and/or money by accepting the therapy being offered.

Chapter VI

MALPRACTICE AND OTHER TORTS

Persons within our society have an obligation, which is recognized by courts, to not act in ways that will adversely affect the physical condition, mental condition, reputation, or property of those with whom they directly or indirectly interact. They have this obligation *regardless* of whether there are laws that specifically prohibit their actions. Ignoring this obligation can result in their being sued for committing a *tort* by a person who was adversely affected by the act. If a clinician, for example, were to use corporal punishment to discipline a child without parental permission, the child's parents could sue the clinician for the tort of *battery.* Or if the use of response-contingent "time out" caused a child a great deal of mental distress, the child's parents could sue the clinician for the tort of *infliction of mental distress.* Or if a clinician told potential patients of a practitioner that he or she was incompetent or unethical, the practitioner could sue the clinician for the tort of *slander.* Or if you entered someone's office without permission, the person could sue you for the tort of *trespass.* Whether the person initiating any of these suits (i.e., the plaintiff) would be likely to win would be determined by several factors. These are discussed elsewhere in this chapter.

My objective in this chapter is to acquaint you with the law of torts, particularly as it relates to clinical practice in speech-language pathology and audiology. I shall begin by describing some of the basic characteristics of torts. Next, I will describe some types of torts that can be professionally relevant, including the negligence tort of *malpractice.* Finally, we will consider how a speech-language pathologist or audiologist might function so as to minimize the probability of becoming involved in tort-related litigation. Malpractice and other types of insurance that offer some protection if sued for committing a tort will be discussed.

WHAT IS A TORT?

There appears to be almost universal agreement among writers of books on torts that the term "tort" is a difficult one to define in a completely (or even almost completely) satisfactory manner (Prosser, 1971). One reason is that some of the acts that the courts have classified as torts seem to have little in common. Another reason is that the courts through their decisions (see Chapter 2 for a discussion of the lawmaking function of the courts) have classified acts they had not previously classified as torts as includable in this category. Some of these would not have been predictable from definitions of the term "tort" in existence at the time (Prosser, 1971).

Courts create torts: Acts become torts when they are classified as such by the courts. This may be one reason why it has been difficult to arrive at a satisfactory definition of the term "tort." Existing definitions appear to have been based, at least in part, on explanations that judges have included in their decisions for why they have classified the acts as torts. However, the reasons given may not have been their real ones for doing so.

While existing definitions of the term "tort" are not completely satisfactory, they do shed some light on the characteristics of acts that the courts have given permission to be assigned to this category. The following partial definitions that have been suggested for the term "tort" are helpful in understanding this concept:

1. A private or civil wrong or injury. A wrong independent of contract (Black, 1968, p. 1660).
2. A legal wrong committed upon the person or property independent of contract. It may be either (1) a direct invasion of some legal right of the individual; (2) the infraction of some public duty by which special damage accrues to the individual; (3) the violation of some private obligation by which like damage accrues to the individual. In the former case, no special damage is necessary to entitle the party to recover. In the two latter cases, such damage is necessary (Black, 1968, pp. 1660–1661).
3. A tort is a breach of a duty (other than a contractual or quasi-contractual duty) which gives rise to an action for damages (Prosser, 1971, p. 1).
4. A tort is an act or omission which unlawfully violates a person's right created by the law, and for which the appropriate remedy is a common law action for damages by the injured person (Prosser, 1971, p. 2).
5. Broadly speaking, a tort is a civil wrong, other than breach of contract,

for which the court will provide a remedy in the form of an action for damages (Prosser, 1971, p. 2).

6. It might be possible to define a tort by enumerating the things it is not. It is not a crime, it is not breach of contract, it is not necessarily concerned with property rights or problems of government, but it is the occupant of a large residuary field remaining if these are taken out of the law (Prosser, 1971, p. 2).

7. Included under the head of torts are a miscellaneous group of civil wrongs, ranging from simple, direct interference with person, such as assault, battery and false imprisonment, or with property, as in the case of trespass or conversion, up through various forms of negligence, to disturbances of intangible interests, such as those in good reputation, or commercial or social advantage. These wrongs have little in common and appear at first glance to be entirely unrelated to one another ... and it is not easy to discover any general principle upon which they may all be based, unless it is the obvious one that *injuries are to be compensated and anti-social behavior is to be discouraged* [italics mine] (Prosser, 1971, p. 3).

8. ... the function and purpose of the law of torts. Contract liability is imposed by the law for the protection of a single, limited interest, that of having the promises of others performed. Quasi-contractual liability is created for the prevention of unjust enrichment of one man at the expense of another, and the restitution of benefits which in good conscience belong to the plaintiff. The criminal law is concerned with the protection of interests common to the public at large, as they are represented by the entity which we call the state; and it accomplishes its ends by exacting a penalty from the wrongdoer. *There remains a body of law which is directed toward the compensation of individuals, rather than the public, for losses which they have suffered in respect of all their legally recognized interests, rather than one interest only, where the law considers that compensation is required* [italics mine]. This is the law of torts (Prosser, 1971, pp. 5–6).

9. The entire history of the development of tort law shows a continuous tendency to recognize as worthy of legal protection interests which previously were not protected at all. ... It is altogether unlikely that this tendency to give protection to hitherto unprotected interests and to extend a greater protection to those now frequently protected has ceased (*Restatement of the Law: Torts*, 1965–1979, Section 1).

Several general characteristics of torts are indicated in these definitions. First, torts are *civil wrongs* rather than criminal wrongs. They are not crimes. They are wrongs against individuals rather than against society.

Hence, in a lawsuit involving a tort the plaintiff is a person, or group of persons, rather than a governmental unit (e.g., the state).

A second characteristic of a tort is that it is a civil wrong for which a court will provide a *remedy*. The remedy may be an award of money (i.e., damages) to compensate the injured party for the wrong done to him or her, or an order to the defendant to cease doing whatever he or she is doing that is causing the plaintiff to be wronged (i.e., an injunction), or something else.

The willingness of the court to provide a remedy for some civil wrongs (such as libel and negligence) is well established. For others, it may be necessary to initiate a suit to establish the courts' willingness to provide a remedy—that is, to establish their willingness to classify the type of wrong done to the plaintiff as a tort.

A third characteristic of a tort is that it is a civil wrong that *does not directly involve the breach of a contract.* The breach of a contract is a civil wrong resulting from the failure of a person to do what he or she *voluntarily* promised to do. (See Chapter 5 for further information about contracts.) The same act performed by a person who had *not* voluntarily agreed to refrain from doing it (by entering into a contract) probably would not be regarded by a court as a civil wrong (assuming that a judge would not regard it as a tort). On the other hand, one is *expected* by society to refrain from engaging in acts that can cause injury to others. Hence, the breach of a contract differs from a tort in that the former involves the breaking of a promise that one has made *voluntarily* to a *specific person* (or a relatively small group of persons) and the latter involves the breaking of a promise that one was *required by "law" to make to all persons* with whom one interacts (e.g., not to do something intentionally that can cause them injury).

A fourth characteristic of a tort is that it results from *interference with the realization of a legally protected desire.* The realization of certain desires is regarded by the courts to be of such social importance that they are obliged to discourage persons from thwarting them. They do this by imposing *liability* (e.g., damages) on those who thwart or set up roadblocks that interfere with the realization of these desires either *intentionally* or through *negligence*.

What *types of desires* have the courts been willing to protect from being thwarted? There are many (see the multivolume work, *Restatement of the Law: Torts*, 1965–1979), including the following:

1. The desire for *bodily security* — the desire not to be physically harmed or even being touched by another without your permission, either intentionally or through negligence (e.g., malpractice).
2. The desire for a *reputation* that is commensurate with your behavior — the desire not to have your reputation damaged by someone's saying or writing something about you that is not true.
3. The desire for your *property* to be secure — the desire for your property not to be damaged, used, or even touched by another without your permission, either intentionally or through negligence.
4. The desire for your *mental state* to be secure — the desire not to have your intellectual or emotional status harmed by another, either intentionally or through negligence.

Some torts that can result from these types of desires being thwarted are described in the next section of this chapter.

TYPES OF TORTS

Most actions that are classifiable as torts can be assigned to one of the following three categories: negligence torts, intentional torts, or strict liability (see Figure 6.1). This section describes some professionally relevant torts that are representative of those in each category.

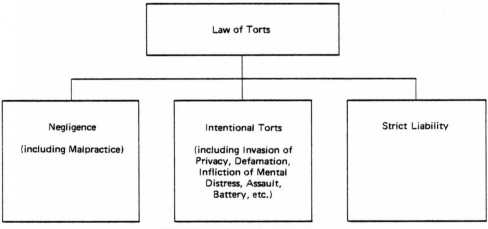

FIGURE 6.1 Classification of torts.

Negligence Torts

Negligence torts involve carelessness that injures (or harms) others. However, not all accidents are regarded by the courts as torts of negligence. In order for an accident to be so regarded, the following four conditions must be met:

The actor [i.e., the person causing the accident] is liable for an invasion of an interest of another, if:

(a) the interest invaded is protected against unintentional invasion, and

(b) the conduct of the actor is negligent with respect to the other, or to a class of persons within which he is included, and

(c) the actor's conduct is a legal cause of the invasion, and

(d) the other has not conducted himself as to disable himself from bringing an action for an invasion. (*Restatement of the Law: Torts,* 1965–1979, Section 281)

The first and second conditions must be met for the conduct of a person who is responsible for an accident to be regarded as negligent by the courts. The third and fourth conditions must be met before a court probably would be willing to award damages for negligent conduct, once it had been established that it had occurred. If the first two conditions were met but not the third and fourth, the court might agree that the actor's conduct was negligent but would not award damages. Hence, the attorney for a defendant in a malpractice suit may attempt to prove that the third and/or fourth condition was not met and, for this reason, damages should not be awarded to the plaintiff.

What interests are protected by the courts against *unintentional* invasion? The courts have been willing to protect a number of interests against unintentional invasion by reason of carelessness. The following excerpts from the authoritative *Restatement of the Law: Torts* (1965–1979) indicates some of the types of negligent acts against which the courts have been willing to offer protection:

1. . . . acts which are generally regarded as reasonably safe if properly done, the only danger involved in them lying in the chance that the actor may be inattentive, incompetent, or unskillful or that he may fail to make adequate preparation or give adequate warning [Section 297]. When an act is negligent only if done without reasonable care, the care which the actor is required to exercise to avoid being negligent in the doing of the act is that which a *reasonable man* [italics mine] in his

position, with his information and competence, would recognize as necessary to prevent the act from creating an unreasonable risk of harm to another [Section 298].

(a) An act may be negligent if it is done without the competence which a *reasonable man* [italics mine] in the position of the actor would recognize as necessary to prevent it creating an unreasonable risk of harm to another [Section 299]. Unless he represents that he has greater or less skill or knowledge, one who undertakes to render services in the practice of a profession or trade is required to exercise the skill and knowledge normally possessed by members of that profession or trade in good standing in similar communities [Section 299A].

(b) When an act is negligent when done without reasonable preparation, the actor, to avoid being negligent, is required to make the preparation which a *reasonable man* [italics mine] in his position would recognize as necessary to prevent the act from creating an unreasonable risk of harm to another [Section 300].

2. An act may be negligent if the actor attempts to prevent, or realizes or should realize that it is likely to prevent, another or a third person from taking action which the actor realizes or should realize is necessary for the aid or protection of the other [Section 305]. [Beginning voice therapy before having a client's vocal folds checked for pathology by an otolaryngologist may be viewed by a court as such an act.]

3. An act may be negligent, as creating an unreasonable risk of bodily harm to another, if the actor intends to subject, or realizes or should realize that his act involves an unreasonable risk of subjecting, the other to an emotional disturbance of such a character as to be likely to result in illness or other bodily harm [Section 306].

4. It is negligence to use an instrumentality, whether a human being or a thing, which the actor knows or should know to be so incompetent, inappropriate, or defective, that its use involves an unreasonable risk of harm to others [Section 307]. [The use of students in training to provide clinical services without adequate supervision may be viewed by the courts as this type of negligent act.]

For further information about the types of negligent acts referred to in these excerpts as well as other types of negligent acts for which courts have been willing to provide a remedy, see Chapters 12 through 19 in *Restatement of the Law: Torts* (1965–1979), Bebout's (1986) paper, "The malpractice storm," Feuer's (1990) book, *Medical Malpractice Law*, Kooper and Sullivan's chapter, "Professional liability: Management and prevention (1986), and Rowland's (1988) paper, "Malpractice in audiology and speech-language pathology."

What standard do the courts use to judge whether the conduct of an actor was negligent? The standard, which is referred to in several of these excerpts, is that of the hypothetical *reasonable man.* A person who does not take the precautions that *a reasonable man in the same position* would be expected to take in order to avoid harming others is likely to be regarded as negligent by a court if someone is harmed by the act: "Unless the actor is a child, the standard to which he must conform to avoid being negligent is that of a reasonable man under like circumstances" (*Restatement of the Law: Torts,* Section 283).

If the standard of conduct to which you must conform to avoid being negligent is that of a reasonable man under like circumstances, you should be aware of the *qualities* that the courts ascribe to their hypothetical reasonable man. These are summarized as follows in Section 283 of the *Restatement of the Law: Torts:*

> The words "reasonable man" denote a person exercising those qualities of attention, knowledge, intelligence, and judgment which society requires of its members for the protection of their own interests and the interests of others. It enables those who are to determine whether the actor's conduct is such as to subject him to liability for harm caused thereby, to express their judgment in terms of the conduct of a human being. The fact that this judgment is personified in a "man" calls attention to the necessity of taking into account the fallibility of human beings.

Deciding whether a person's conduct in a particular situation conforms to what would be expected from a reasonable man in like circumstances may not be easy because it may be unclear how a reasonable man would conduct himself. The attorney for the defendant in a negligence suit is likely to attempt to convince the judge and jury that his or her client's conduct conformed to that of the hypothetical reasonable man and, hence, the *second* of the four conditions that must be satisfied before a court is supposed to award damages for negligence has not been met.

The *third condition* that has to be met before an accident is likely to be regarded by a court as resulting from negligence is that the actor's (defendant's) conduct be the *legal cause* of the harm to the plaintiff. Thus, it is not enough to be able to demonstrate that you were harmed because of the negligence of another. You also have to demonstrate that the negligent act that caused the harm is one for which the courts have been willing to award damages and, hence, has been recognized as a legal cause.

What causes have the courts recognized as legal causes? According to Section 431 of the *Restatement of the Law: Torts:*

The actor's negligent conduct is a legal cause of harm to another if

(a) his conduct is a *substantial factor* [italics mine] in bringing about the harm, and

(b) there is no rule of law relieving the actor from liability because of the manner in which his negligence has resulted in harm.

The defendant's conduct is likely to be viewed as a substantial factor in bringing about the plaintiff's harm if a *reasonable man* would be likely to regard it as such. The attorney for the defendant may attempt to demonstrate that while his or her conduct was negligent, it would not be regarded by the hypothetical reasonable man as being the real cause of the harm done to the plaintiff. If the attorney is successful, the plaintiff would be unlikely to be awarded damages.

A defendant can be relieved of liability for a particular negligent act if there is a *rule of law* that relieves persons from negligence liability for that act. A physician, for example, may be relieved from negligence liability for complications arising from an emergency tracheotomy performed on a person who probably would have died otherwise if there is a law that prevents physicians from being sued for harm resulting from such emergency procedures.

The *fourth and final condition* that must be met before a court is likely to award damages for negligence is that the plaintiff must have conducted himself or herself in a manner that would not disqualify him or her from suing for damages. A plaintiff can be disqualified by acting in a manner that is *below the standard of conduct* that a reasonable man would expect of someone for their own protection. Plaintiffs who did so would be contributing to the negligence that caused them to be harmed. In some states, if a defendant can prove *contributory negligence* on the part of the plaintiff, this will bar the plaintiff from receiving damages; in other states, contributory negligence does not disqualify the plaintiff from being awarded damages but is considered by the court when deciding the amount of damages to award (*Restatement of the Law: Torts,* 1965–1979, Chapter 17).

What constitutes contributory negligence on the part of a plaintiff? According to the *Restatement of the Law: Torts* (Sections 463 & 464), contributory negligence can be defined as follows:

> Contributory negligence is conduct on the part of the plaintiff which falls below the standard to which he should conform for his own protection, and which is a legally contributing cause co-operating with the negligence of the defendant in bringing about the plaintiff's harm. . . . Unless the actor is a child or an insane person, the standard of conduct to which he must conform for his own protection is that of the *reasonable man under like circumstances.*

The attorney for the defendant in a negligence suit may attempt to prove that the plaintiff did not protect himself or herself as well as a *reasonable man* would be expected to under the circumstances and, hence, the plaintiff was negligent.

We have considered thus far the general conditions that must be met before an act causing harm to another is likely to be regarded by the courts as a negligence tort. The remainder of this section deals with the type of negligence tort that probably is of most concern to speech-language pathologists and audiologists—*malpractice.*

What constitutes malpractice? In general, any type of negligent conduct by a professional that causes his or her patient (client) to be harmed either physically or mentally may be viewed by a court as constituting malpractice. As applied to health care professionals,

> the term means, generally, professional misconduct toward a patient which is considered reprehensible either because being immoral in itself or because being contrary to law or expressly forbidden by law.
>
> In a more specific sense it means bad, wrong, or injudicious treatment of a patient, professionally and in respect to the particular disease or injury, resulting in injury, unnecessary suffering, or death of the patient, and proceeding from ignorance, carelessness, want of proper professional skills, disregard of established rules or principles, neglect, or a malicious or criminal intent (Black, 1968, p. 1111).

Society expects professionals, such as speech-language pathologists and audiologists, to exercise reasonable care and to possess a standard minimum of special knowledge and ability (Prosser, 1971). The standard minimum ordinarily is that specified in the requirements for the license or certification required for practicing the profession.

The defendants in the majority of malpractice suits involving health care professionals have been physicians. However, practitioners in almost every health care field, including speech-language pathology and audiology, have been defendants in such suits (Miller, 1983; Miller & Lubinski, 1986). Because of the risk of being ruined financially by a malpractice suit, almost all health care professionals have malpractice insurance. Even if a professional wins such a suit, the legal fees for defending himself or herself can be quite high (see Liability lawsuits present danger to qualified professionals, says official, 1985). Speech-language pathologists and audiologists who are employed by school systems, hospitals, or other institutions *usually* are provided malpractice insurance coverage by their employer. Those who are engaged in private practice (either full or part time), however, have to arrange for their own malpractice insurance. For the names of companies that offer it, contact the American Speech-Language-Hearing Association.

What types of conduct by a speech-language pathologist or audiologist could lead to a malpractice suit? There are a number of scenarios that could lead to such a suit including the following:

1. A speech-language pathologist accepts for voice therapy a person who has a hoarse voice and does not insist that he be seen by an otolaryngologist for a laryngeal examination. The person discovers six months later that his hoarseness resulted from laryngeal cancer. He claims that he was harmed because the condition was not diagnosed earlier and that this was due to the speech-language pathologists negligence in not insisting on his having a laryngeal examination before therapy was begun.

2. A speech-language pathologist administers swallowing therapy to an adult who has been diagnosed as having dysphagia. The clinician does not have suctioning equipment in the room that she (or someone else such as a nurse) can use if the person begins to choke. The client chokes on some food during a therapy session and dies. The family sues the speech-language pathologist claiming that she had been negligent by not having suctioning equipment available in the room while doing the swallowing therapy.

3. An audiologist inserts an impedance probe into a child's ear without first examining the external canal with an otoscope to make certain that there is no object in the canal that could damage the tympanic membrane if pushed against it. The insertion of the probe results in an object being pushed against the membrane and damaging it. The family sues the audiologist claiming that he or she has been negligent by not examining the canal before inserting the probe.

4. An audiologist participates in the initial diagnosis of deafness in a young child. Later, the parents produce a second child who is also deaf. The parents sue the audiologist claiming that he was negligent

by failing to advise them to obtain genetic counseling following the diagnosis of deafness in the first child.

5. A two-year-old child swallowed the battery of a hearing aid that had been prescribed by an audiologist. Surgery was necessary to remove the battery. The parents sue the audiologist claiming that he was negligent by not warning them about the possibility of this occurring.

For additional scenarios relevant to our profession, see Kramer and Armbruster (1982) Lowe (1988), and Rowland (1988).

Intentional Torts

Intentional torts result from acts that are *intended* to injure or harm others and/or are morally wrong. They differ from negligence torts in that the harm done to a person is not due to carelessness. If I told someone that a fellow professional is a quack, my *intent* probably would have been to damage his or her reputation and, thereby, discourage people from utilizing his or her services. If the person sued me and I was unable to prove that he or she is not at least a minimally competent practitioner, the court would be likely to award him damages for being slandered.

The word *intent,* as used in this context, denotes the actor's awareness that his or her act is likely to have certain consequences. According to Section 8A of the *Restatement of the Law: Torts,*

> All consequences which the actor desires to bring about are intended. . . . Intent is not, however, limited to consequences which are desired. If the actor knows that the consequences are certain, or substantially certain, to result from his act, and still goes ahead, he is treated by the law as if he had in fact desired to produce the result. As the probability that the consequences will follow decreases, and becomes less than substantial certainty, the actor's conduct loses the character of intent, and becomes mere recklessness. . . . As the probability decreases further, and amounts only to a risk that the result will follow, it becomes ordinary negligence.

Thus, people can be held accountable not only for desired consequences of their acts, but also for others that they know are likely to occur.

What *types of acts* are the courts likely to classify as intentional torts? Some of those that can be professionally relevant are described briefly in the paragraphs which follow. For further information about intentional torts, see Prosser (1971) and *Restatement of the Law: Torts* (1965–1979).

Invasion of Privacy. It has been recognized by the courts that people have a right to privacy—a right to be let alone. Interference with this right can result in the tort *invasion of privacy*. Such interference can take many forms, several of which are particularly relevant professionally.

It can be regarded as interference with clients' rights to privacy to *release information* about them from their clinic folder without their written consent, to *use photographs* of them in clinic promotional material without written consent, to write about them in published case studies *in a manner that makes them recognizable* without such consent, or to allow anyone to *view their clinic sessions from behind a one-way mirror* without it. Several forms that can be used for securing a client's written consent are in Appendix A.

Defamation. If someone says or writes something *false and malicious* about you that injures your reputation, you *may be successful* if you sue that person for the tort of libel or of slander. If the false and malicious statements were communicated in *written or printed* form, you ordinarily would sue for *libel;* if they were communicated in *oral* form, you ordinarily would sue for *slander.* The law in this area is quite complex, and you would have to consult with an attorney to determine whether the courts would be likely to award you *sufficient damages* to make a suit for defamation (i.e., slander or libel) worthwhile. You could conceivably win a defamation suit and be awarded only *nominal damages* — for example, one dollar.

Not all statements which have been made about you that you regard as being false and malicious would be likely to be viewed by the courts as being libelous or slanderous. Under what circumstances are they apt to be so viewed? According to Prosser,

> defamation is — that which tends to injure "reputation" in the popular sense; to diminish the esteem, respect, goodwill or confidence in which the plaintiff is held, or to excite adverse, derogatory or unpleasant feelings or opinions against him. It necessarily, however, involves the idea of *disgrace* [italics mine] (1971, p. 729).

While the statement that an audiologist is sympathetic to the use of sign rather than speech by deaf persons is likely to elicit negative feelings against him or her in the minds of those who are against their use of sign and may even diminish the audiologist in their esteem, a court would be unlikely to consider it defamatory. A *reasonable man* would be unlikely to consider that it reflects upon the audiologist's character and, hence, would cause him or her to be disgraced. On the other hand, a statement that the audiologist is *unethical* would be likely to be viewed by a court as defamatory since a reasonable man would be likely to conclude that it reflects on the audiologist's character and, hence, could cause him or her to be disgraced.

A professional's reputation determines to a considerable extent how successfully he or she is likely to be financially and otherwise. Therefore, the courts have recognized that they have a special responsibility to protect professionals against false and malicious statements about their capacity and professional conduct. Speech-language pathologists and audiologists not only risk lawsuits by making false and malicious statements about other professionals, but they also violate the Code of Ethics of the American Speech-Language-Hearing Association (see Chapter 3 and Appendix D).

Infliction of Mental Distress. If someone *purposely* said and/or did something (or is saying and/or doing something) that caused you to become *severely* emotionally disturbed, or mentally disturbed, you could attempt to obtain relief from a court. The relief you would seek might be an *injunction* that would order the person to stop saying or doing what is causing you to be mentally distressed or it might be *damages* to compensate you for the detrimental effects that the mental distress has produced.

The word "severely" was italicized in the preceding paragraph to indicate that the courts are unlikely to compensate you for most things people are apt to say or do that make you upset. The courts assume that a *reasonable man* should be able to keep from becoming overly upset by most potentially irritating things that people say or do. Also if the courts were willing to award damages for insults and most other things people do that upset us, there probably would be so many lawsuits that the civil courts would become hopelessly bogged down.

What types of stress-inducing conduct are the courts likely to compensate you for? According to Section 46 of the *Restatement of the Law: Torts:*

> one who by extreme and outrageous conduct intentionally or recklessly causes severe emotional distress to another is subject to liability for such emotional distress, and if bodily harm to the other results from it, for such bodily harm.

Hence, for the conduct that caused your emotional distress to be compensable, it would have to be such that the hypothetical reasonable man would view it as *extreme and outrageous*. The courts are likely to consider the following comment from Section 46 of the *Restatement of the*

Law: Torts as a guideline when deciding whether conduct has been extreme and outrageous:

> *Extreme and outrageous conduct.* The cases thus far decided have found liability only where the defendant's conduct has been extreme and outrageous. It has not been enough that the defendant has acted with an intent which is tortious or even criminal, or that he has intended to inflict emotional distress, or even that his conduct has been characterized by "malice," or a degree of aggravation which would entitle the plaintiff to punitive damages for another tort. Liability has been found only where the conduct has been so outrageous in character, and so extreme in degree, as to go beyond all possible bounds of decency, and to be regarded as atrocious, and utterly intolerable in a civilized community. Generally, the case is one in which the recitation of the facts to an *average member of the community* [italics mine] would arouse his resentment against the actor, and lead him to exclaim, "Outrageous!"

One technique that some speech-language pathologists and audiologists have used with communicatively handicapped children and adults that could be viewed by the average member of the community as extreme and outrageous is the use of a response-contingent punisher, such as electric shock. The average member of your community (whose views would reflect the attitudes of most juries) is likely to look upon giving a handicapped child electric shocks as outrageous. It is essential, therefore, that written consent be obtained from clients or their families before using any intervention strategy that could be viewed by "the average member of your community" in this manner. The *rationale* for using the approach and the *risks* involved should be explained to the client's family and possibly to the client so that the written consent procured is likely to be looked upon by a court as being *informed consent* (see Chapter 10).

Assault. If others by their actions and/or words caused you to become *apprehensive* about being harmed by them (that is, if they threaten to harm you), you can sue them for the tort of assault. Assault does not involve actual undesired physical contact, only the *threat* of such contact. This tort is actually a special case of *infliction of mental distress* —the mental distress being caused by a threat of physical harm.

Battery. If someone *intentionally touched you without your permission* (even if the contact resulted in no physical injury such as would ordinarily be the case for a kiss), you could sue them for the tort of battery. The courts will protect your right to freedom from *intentional and unpermitted physical contacts* (Prosser, 1971).

This tort differs from assault in that there is actual physical contact. If someone both made you apprehensive about being physically harmed and intentionally physically touched you, you could sue them for both *assault and battery.*

Since plaintiffs in a suit for battery do not have to prove that they were physically harmed—only that they were touched without permission—this tort could have implications for clinicians. Touching a client lightly on the arm without permission could lead to being sued for battery as could removal of his or her hearing aid without permission (Rowland, 1988). While few clients are likely to even consider initiating such a suit, a clinician should be aware of the possibility and refrain from touching a client who seems like the "suing kind." Obviously such a suit (whether or not it had any merit) could seriously damage a clinician's reputation.

Strict Liability

In both negligence torts and intentional torts, a plaintiff is awarded damages because the conduct of the defendant was in some way *faulty.* When suing for these types of torts, the plaintiff must establish that the negligence or purposeful conduct of the defendant was responsible for the harm done to him or her before a court will award damages.

In some cases, the fact that the plaintiff was harmed by the defendant will be sufficient to cause the court to award the plaintiff damages. According to Prosser,

> . . . the last hundred years have witnessed the overthrow of the doctrine of "never any liability without fault," even in the legal sense of departure from reasonable standards of conduct. It has seen a general acceptance of the principle that in some cases the defendant may be held liable, although he is not only charged with no moral wrongdoing, but has not even departed in any way from a reasonable standard of intent or care. . . . This new policy frequently has found expression when the defendant's activity is unusual and abnormal in the community, and the danger which it threatens to others is unduly great—and particularly where the danger will be great even though the enterprise is conducted with every possible precaution (1971, p. 494).

Thus, an industrial firm could be held responsible for certain hearing losses of its employees because they are exposed to extremely high levels of noise even though the firm took "every possible precaution."

TORT LITIGATION AND THE CLINICIAN

Speech-language pathologists and audiologists, like practitioners in other health-related professions, run risk of becoming involved in tort-related litigation as a defendant. Since such litigation can have a disastrous impact on both the practitioners' finances and their reputations, they should do everything they can to minimize the risk. They can do this by increasing their awareness of events that can occur in their interactions with clients and client's families that could lead to such litigation and then taking appropriate precautions. If they are uncertain about whether the precautions they are taking are adequate, they would be wise to consult with an attorney.

The risk of being sued for a tort can be minimized, but it cannot be eliminated entirely. It is important, therefore, to have adequate *professional liability insurance* (see Miller, 1983; Miller & Libinski, 1986). It usually will be provided by your employer unless your relationship to him or her is one of *independent contractor* (see Chapter 9). If it is not provided by your employer or you are in private practice, contact the American Speech-Language-Association for information about vendors.

Chapter VII

RECORDS MANAGEMENT

A ll speech-language pathologists and audiologists keep various types of records, including information about persons who have received or are receiving clinical services. Such information may be recorded on sheets of paper, on audiotape or videotape, or on photographic film (such as microfilm), and/or it may be stored in a computer. Although the needs of the clinician are the primary determiners of what information is collected and how it is used, the law places restrictions and obligations (directly and indirectly) on both of these. In this chapter we will consider some aspects of records management on which there are such restrictions and obligations. Since interpretations of the laws that impose them are likely to change from time to time because of new legislation and court decisions (see the discussion of *stare decisis* in Chapter 2), the specific restrictions and obligations that were imposed when this chapter was written are not described in detail. The details of a restriction or obligation are more likely to change than the restriction or obligation itself.

What laws govern the management of clinical records of speech-language pathologists and audiologists is determined, at least partially, by the type of setting in which they are working. If they are working in an *educational* setting—such as a public school or a college—the relevant laws will be those for the management of school records. If they are working in a *medical* setting—such as a hospital or nursing home—the relevant laws will be those for the management of medical records. Thus, speech-language pathologists and audiologists can obtain up-to-date information about at least some of the relevant laws by studying guidelines for records management in the type of setting in which they are employed.

We shall begin by considering the kinds of clinical information, or data, that the courts are likely to regard as records. We then shall consider some aspects of records management for which there are legal restrictions and obligations, including record content and documentation, record storage and confidentiality, ownership of records, access of clients and their families to records, correcting errors in records, record retention and statutes of limitation, transfer of information at the request of the client or client's family, requests for information by someone other than the client or client's family, and the use of client records for clinical research. My objective here is to highlight aspects of records management about which you should be concerned rather than provide specific guidelines. An attorney who is retained by your employer should be able to provide such guidelines.

KINDS OF DATA REGARDED BY THE COURTS AS BEING PART OF A CLINIC RECORD

A record is *an account of what has been done* (Black, 1968). Although such an account usually is written or printed on sheets of paper or stored in a computer, it may be recorded on microfilm or conveyed, at least partially, by means of recordings (e.g., pretherapy and posttherapy speech samples) or photographs (e.g., x-rays films).

Almost any kind of data that helps to tell the story of what was done to a person while he or she was receiving clinical services at a particular institution (e.g., a public school or a hospital) may be regarded by a court as being a part of his or her clinic record and, hence, can be requested (by a court order or *subpoena*) as evidence. Included here would be evaluation and progress reports, case histories, clinician's notes about what transpired during particular sessions and telephone conversations, forms on which test results are recorded, payments records for services, and pretherapy and posttherapy tapes.

SOME ASPECTS OF CLINICAL RECORDS MANAGEMENT ON WHICH THERE ARE LEGAL RESTRICTIONS AND OBLIGATIONS

The clinical record systems maintained by speech-language pathologists and audiologists are required by law to be managed in certain ways. Some of the means through which the law imposes restrictions and obligations on the management of such systems will be indicated in this section.

Record Content and Documentation

The specific types of information that speech-language pathologists and audiologists are expected to collect on the persons to whom they provide clinical services is partially determined by regulations promulgated by administrative agencies, including state departments of public instruction and federal agencies such as the Social Security Administration (which administers the Medicare and Medicaid programs). These agencies influence record content by demanding certain types of *documentation* on those persons for whose clinical services they are at least partially paying.

If a clinician does not collect the information an agency requires for documenting what has been done to a client, he or she will obviously be unable to provide the documentation, which could result, for example, in the employer's not being paid for the services. This would not endear the clinician to his or her employer, regardless of whether the institution was a public school, hospital, or other clinical facility. Clinicians would be wise, therefore, to check periodically with their administrators to make certain that they are collecting all of the information required for documenting their services and for the various other purposes for which documentation is needed.

Record Storage and Confidentiality

One factor that a speech-language pathologist or audiologist must take into consideration when establishing a clinical record storage system is that of providing adequate safeguards for keeping the information stored in it confidential. It has been recognized since ancient times (see the *Oath of Hippocrates*, which is reproduced in Chapter 3) that information that a clinician learns about a patient is confidential and *ordinarily* not to be divulged to anyone without the patient's permission. This obligation is recognized in the current (1991) version of the Code of Ethics of the American Speech-Language-Hearing Association (see Appendix D):

> Individuals must not reveal to unauthorized persons any professional or personal information obtained from the person served professionally, unless required by law or unless necessary to protect the welfare of the person or the community.

Obviously, this prohibition applied to *both* written and oral communication. Furthermore, since failure to keep information confidential can harm a client's *reputation*, it can result in a clinician being sued for *defamation* — i.e., for *libel* if the information is communicated in a report (or other document) or for *slander* if it is communicated orally (Feuer, 1990). (See Chapter 6 for descriptions of these torts.)

One of the first decisions that has to be made when designing confidentiality safeguards for a clinical record system is to decide who is authorized to see the records. Persons who would be so authorized would include the client's clinician and others whom the client gave permission in writing to see the records. They also would include those associated with the institution whom our hypothetical reasonable man would regard as having a good reason for seeing them — for example, personnel responsible for billing.

Another group who may have good reason to see clients' records are students in training who are observing evaluation and therapy sessions. Some such observation is required for ASHA certificates of clinical competence in both speech-language pathology and audiology. This group is of particular concern to administrators of university speech and hearing clinics. It is common practice in many such clinics to allow undergraduates to see the folders of persons whose evaluation or therapy sessions they are observing. These folders can contain information that our hypothetical reasonable man would not feel such students need to see (e.g., billing information). Clinicians would be wise, therefore, to limit the information to which students are given access to that to which they need to have access to understand what they are observing. Clinicians also would be wise to obtain their clients' (and/or their clients' families') written permission to make this information available to student observers.

A third group that may have good reason to see clients' records are clinical researchers, possibly ones from institutions other than those at which they were treated (Sieber, 1989; Weil & Hollander, 1990). If such researchers are from institutions at which they were treated, they may or may not have been the ones who treated them. The data for much speech-language pathology and audiology clinical research has come, in whole or part, from clients' records.

To assist both in preserving the confidentiality of client's records and in documenting who had access to them, the procedures should require persons who wish to see records to sign a dated form and fill in their reasons for wanting access to the records. This procedure would assist in preserving the confidentiality of records by discouraging viewing by persons who do not have a legitimate reason for doing so. It would also provide the data necessary for documenting who had had access to particular records if this information is requested by a court.

For further information about legal aspects of record storage and confidentiality, see Annas (1975, Chapters 10 and 11); Hayt, Hayt, and Groeschel (1972, Chapter 47); and Levine and Cary (1977, Chapter 10).

Ownership of Records

Do a client's records legally belong to the client or to the institution that created them for reporting what was done? The answer to this question has implications for several issues, one of which is a person's right to see his or her records.

In most, if not all, employment situations in which speech-language pathologists and audiologists are likely to find themselves the courts are likely to look upon client records as belonging to the institution. The laws of all 50 states, for example, recognize that a patient's hospital records are the property of the hospital (Annas, 1975).

While the institution owns a person's treatment record, it cannot deny the person access to it. As Annas has stated in the context of hospital records:

> Although the hospital is the owner of the record by virtue of custom, and owns the paper on which the record is printed [or the computer in whose memory the record is stored], this still does not mean that it can do whatever it wants with the record. Indeed, there is case authority establishing that while the hospital has a property right in the record, the patient has a property right in the information contained in the record and cannot be denied access to that information (1975, pp. 114–115).

The question of a patient's right to have access to his or her own records is dealt with further in the next section.

Access of Clients and Their Families to Records

Clinicians providing speech-language pathology or audiology services in either an educational or medical setting are required by law to show their clients their diagnostic and treatment records if they ask to see them in the appropriate manner. For those providing these services in an educational setting, the law with which they should be familiar is the Amendment to the Family Educational Rights and Privacy Act (known as the *Buckley Amendment*), which was passed by the Congress in 1974. This amendment guarantees the parents of students the right to examine their children's school records. According to Levine and Cary:

> The major provisions of the law require schools to provide parents of students access to any official records directly relating to their children and an opportunity to a hearing to challenge such records on the grounds that they are inaccurate, misleading or otherwise inappropriate (1977, p. 110).

This amendment also guarantees students who are over the age of eighteen or attending any postsecondary school the right to examine their own school records. Obviously, any records that public school speech-language pathologists keep on the children they are serving are a part of their school records and, hence, subject to the Buckley Amendment.

The procedure that clients or their families would follow to see their records if they received speech, language, and/or hearing services in a medical setting would depend upon the state in which they resided. In most states that do not have laws that enable patients to see their medical records, clients or their families can gain access to them by suing the hospital or nursing home involved and having the records subpoenaed for evidence (Annas, 1975, pp. 116–117). The threat of such a lawsuit is sometimes sufficient to motivate an institution to give a client or family access to the records.

Some states have a law that gives patients or their attorneys the right to inspect their hospital records without having to institute a lawsuit under certain circumstances. For example, that of Massachusetts provides that a patient's medical records "may be inspected by the patient to whom they relate ... and a copy shall be furnished upon his request and a payment of a reasonable fee" (Annas, 1975, p. 117).

The fact that the law gives clients access to their clinical records has implications for deciding what should be included in a client's folder or computer database file. You probably should not include anything that you do not want the client or a family member to see. An example of something you may not want to include would be a "negative" evaluational statement about a member of the client's family and his or her relationship to the client (e.g., "The client's mother seems emotionally constricted and does not relate well to him"). If a client or family member saw such a comment, their rapport with the clinician could be adversely affected. In addition, he or she may initiate legal action to have the comment removed from the record.

Correcting Errors in Records

A clinician may feel that some aspect of a client's record is in error and may wish to correct it. Because erasures may create curiosity, if not suspicion about the reason for the change, it would be wise to line out the incorrect data with a single ink line and the add the date of the lining out, the signature (or initials) of the person doing it, and the correct information (Hayt, Hayt, & Groeschel, 1972).

Record Retention and the Statute of Limitations

For how long must a client's clinical records be retained? Legally, this is determined by the *statutes of limitation* for lawsuits involving contracts and torts. A person is given only a limited period of time to initiate a suit for breach of contract or for commission of a tort (such as malpractice). If he or she waits for a longer time than the applicable statute of limitations allows, he or she will lose the suit, regardless of its merits. From this perspective, it does not appear to be necessary to retain the records of inactive clients for longer than ten years. There may, however, be other reasons for doing so—for example, as a data bank for clinical research.

Transfer of Information at the Request of the Client or the Client's Family

Clinicians are often asked by clients or their families to send copies of all or part of their clinic records to other professionals. These professionals may be speech-language pathologists or audiologists or other types of practitioners such as physicians. Such a transfer should not create any legal problems if the client or a close family member (who is legally responsible for him or her) signs an appropriate release of information form (see Appendix A).

Requests for Information by Someone Other Than the Client or the Client's Family

Speech-language pathologists and audiologists occasionally are asked by somebody other than clients or family members to provide information about clients' communicative disorders, or the services they received and their response to them, or their prognosis for further improvement. Persons who might request such information include newspaper and television reporters, employers, insurance companies, government agencies and attorneys. Before responding to such a request you should consult with an attorney about whether to honor it.

Use of Client Records for Research

Speech-language pathologists and audiologists sometimes wish to use information from client's records for research purposes — to answer questions about the symptomatology, etiology, phenomenology, prevalence, diagnosis, or treatment of communicative disorders. For some research purposes, such as an individual case study, an entire record may be used. For others, such as the frequency of occurrence of a particular symptom among persons diagnosed as having a particular communicative disorder, only a relatively small portion of a client's record is likely to be examined and used. A client's consent ordinarily is not necessary to use records for research purposes, particularly if his or her identity is protected. For further information about legal aspects of clinical research, see Chapter. 10.

Chapter VIII

IMPLICATIONS OF COPYRIGHT AND PATENT LAW FOR THE CLINICIAN

Speech-language pathologists and audiologists use various types of printed and audio-visual materials and computer software in their functioning as clinicians. These include diagnostic tests, intervention programs, games, and photographs and drawings designed for eliciting speech and language samples, as well as computer (e.g., word-processing and database) software intended for meeting administrative responsibilities. Clinicians also use various types of devices—both electronic and nonelectronic—when interacting with their clients. Their use of these materials and devices is regulated by copyright and patent laws. These laws also protect the interests of practitioners who develop materials and invent devices for clinical use.

What are copyrights and patents and how do they differ? A copyright can protect the expression of an idea, but not the idea itself. A patent, on the other hand, can protect an idea. These concepts are elaborated upon elsewhere in the chapter.

My objective in this chapter is to acquaint you with those aspects of *property law* dealing with copyrights and patents that are relevant to either (1) the *utilization* of materials and equipment developed by others or (2) the *protection of your interests* in materials and equipment you have developed. I will begin by indicating the objectives of copyright and patent laws. Next, I will describe some aspects of copyright law that are relevant to speech-language pathologists and audiologists. Finally, I will describe some aspects of patent law that could impact on them.

OBJECTIVES OF COPYRIGHT AND PATENT LAW

Our federal government has recognized since its beginnings that authors and inventors should be allowed to profit financially from their creations. This recognition appears to have had its origin in natural law (see

Chapter 2), which would view it as only *fair* that inventors and authors be granted the *exclusive right* to benefit from their creations for a *limited period of time*. The framers of the Constitution, in fact, felt so strongly about the need to protect the right of authors and inventors to profit from their creations that they gave Congress the following power in Article 1, Section 8:

> Congress shall have the power . . . to promote the progress of science and useful arts, by securing for limited times to authors and inventors the exclusive right to their respective writings and discoveries.

The mechanism created by Congress for protecting the rights of authors was the copyright. The corresponding mechanism created for protecting the rights of inventors was the patent.

Copyrights

What is a copyright? It is the right to copy an author's work. The person owning the copyright, who may or may not be the author, has the *exclusive right* for a specified period of time to make and sell copies of the work; hence, he or she holds the *copy right* for the work. The work may be perceivable by vision, audition, touch, or some combination of the three. Works of authorship that are perceivable by vision include books, computer programs, photographs, and drawings. An example of a work of authorship that is perceivable by audition is a "sound" recording on an audiotape cassette or reel, phonograph record, compact disk (CD), or digital audiotape (DAT) cartridge. And an example of a work of authorship that is perceivable by touch is a book printed in Braille. Examples of works of authorship that are perceivable through more than one sense modality are videotape recordings and sound motion pictures.

Copyright laws have two basic objectives, both of which can be inferred from Article 1, Section 8 of the Constitution (quoted earlier in this chapter). The first "is to foster the creation and dissemination of intellectual works for the public welfare" (Dible, 1978, p. 115). These laws "foster the creation and dissemination of intellectual works" by giving the person who publishes them (who may or may not be their author) the opportunity to recoup expenses and possibly make a profit. They do this by making it unlawful for someone else to make copies of the work and sell them for the duration of its copyright. If there were no copyright laws, publishers would be hesitant to invest the money necessary to publish a work because someone else could make copies of the work and possibly sell them at a lower price. They might be able to sell them at a lower price because they would not have some of the production expenses of the original publisher such as copyediting and typesetting. (The assumption here is that they would copy the book photographically.)

The *second objective* of copyright laws "is to give the creators the *reward* [italics mine] due them for their contribution to society" (Dible, 1978, p. 115). They do this in two ways: first, by requiring anyone who copies part of a author's work to indicate the title of the work and the name of its author, and, second, by protecting the author's right to profit financially (e.g., by receiving royalties) from the sale of copies of his or her works. No one is permitted to make and sell copies of an author's work *without his or her permission* for the duration of their copyrights. Presumably, if the author gives somebody, such as a book publisher, permission to make and sell copies of a work, the author will be paid for the privilege (e.g., paid a royalty on each copy sold).

Patents

What is a patent? A patent is "a grant made by the government to an inventor, conveying and securing to him the exclusive right to make, use, and sell his invention for a term of years" (Black, 1968, pp. 1281–1282). This term ordinarily is seventeen years. A patent is not intended to give an inventor the right to make, use, or sell his invention, but (in the language of the 1952 Patent Law) "the right to exclude others from making, using, or selling" the invention. Hence, patents serve the function for inventors that copyrights do for authors. Both "foster the creation and dissemination" of something that contributes to the public welfare (i.e., an invention or a work of authorship). And both "give creators the reward due them for their contributions to society."

PROVISIONS OF COPYRIGHT LAW

The regulations pertaining to copyrights in the United States are contained in the Copyright Act of 1976 (Public Law 94-553). This was the first general revision of U.S. copyright law since 1909. The act became fully effective on January 1, 1978.

The Copyright Act of 1976 is a complex statute. Because of space limitations, I cannot discuss all aspects (or even all major aspects) of it here. The presentation will be limited to aspects that I feel are particularly relevant to speech-language pathologists and audiologists in their roles as clinicians and clinical researchers. The order in which topics are discussed corresponds roughly to the order in which they are mentioned in the statute. (The primary source for this discussion was Dible, 1978, pp. 111–254.)

Duration of Copyright Protection

For works of authorship created after January 1, 1978, the duration of copyright protection is the life of the author plus fifty years after his or her death. For works of more than one author, the fifty year period is measured from the date of the death of the last surviving author. All copyrights run through December 31 of the calendar year in which they expire.

Material That Can Be Copyrighted

The 1976 Copyright Act substitutes the phrase "original works of authorship" for "writings of an author" when designating the material that can be copyrighted. Original works of authorship that can be copyrighted under this act are not limited to those containing written words (which referred to in the statute as "literary works"). These also include: (1) pictorial, graphic, and sculptural works, (2) motion pictures and other audiovisual works, (3) sound recordings, and (4) computer programs.

The category of *literary works* includes any works expressed in "words, numbers, or other verbal or numerical symbols or indicia." While a literary work has to be original in the sense of not being merely a copy of a preexisting work, there is no requirement that it be novel, or ingenuous, or possess esthetic merit. Almost any diagnostic or progress report could be classified for purposes of copyright as a "literary work."

The category of *pictorial, graphic, and sculptural works* includes photographs and drawings (such as those used in diagnostic tests and kits of therapy materials). Photographs and drawings, like literary works, must be original in the sense of not being merely copies of preexisting images, but their novelty, ingenuity, or esthetic merit are not considerations in determining whether they can be copyrighted.

The category of *motion pictures and other audiovisual works* includes videotapes (e.g., videotapes of diagnostic and therapy sessions made by clinicians); the category of *sound recordings* includes phonograph records, audiotapes (e.g., speech and language samples recorded for clinical purposes), compact disks (CDs), and digital audiotape (DAT) cartridges.

Again, novelty, ingenuity, or esthetic merit are not considerations in determining whether a work can be copyrighted.

The category of *computer programs* includes both the code of which programs are comprised and the audiovisual displays that the code produces. These may be copyrighted separately because substantially the same visual and/or audiovisual effect can be achieved by different sets of computer code (Chickering & Hartman, 1987). With computer programs (as with the other categories of material) novelty, ingenuity, or esthetic merit are not considerations in determining whether a work can be copyrighted.

Thus far in this section I have dealt with material that can be copyrighted. What *cannot* be copyrighted? There are six types of materials mentioned in the act that are denied U.S. copyright protection. Three are likely to be of particular interest to speech-language pathologists and audiologists. The first of these is *ideas, methods, systems, and principles.* One of the fundamental principles promulgated by this act is that "copyright does not protect ideas, methods, systems, principles, etc. but rather the *particular manner* [italics mine] in which they are expressed or described" (Dible, 1978, p. 127). Hence, a copyright does not protect a clinician's ideas or methods from being copied; it only protects the particular arrangement of words in which he or she expresses or describes them.

A second type of subject matter that is denied U.S. copyright protection is *blank forms.* According to Dible (1978, p. 127), "Blank forms and similar works designed to record rather than convey information, are not subject to copyright protection." Some of the forms used for recording client's responses to diagnostic tests probably are not protected by copyright for this reason, even though a copyright notice is printed on them. Anyone can place a copyright notice on any work he or she creates, including material that cannot be copyrighted. The copyright notice on such an uncopyrightable test form does serve to discourage others from copying it, simply because most people who use it are not sufficiently familiar with copyright law to know that it cannot be copyrighted.

A third type of subject matter that is denied U.S. copyright protection is *works of the U.S. Government.* According to Dible (1978, p. 128), "works produced for the U.S. Government by its officers and employees *as a part of their official duties* [italics mine] are not subject to U.S. copyright protection." This category does not necessarily include works prepared under a U.S. government contract or grant. The funding agency can decide whether an independent contractor or grantee will be allowed to copyright works that were supported wholly or partially by government funds.

Ownership and Transfer of Rights

The author of a work that was not prepared within the scope of his or her employment is the owner of the copyright on it unless he or she has transferred ownership of the copyright to somebody else. If such a work has more than one author, its authors jointly own the copyright unless they have transferred ownership of the copyright to somebody else.

The copyright to a "work prepared by an employee within the scope of his or her employment" belongs to the employer unless the employer transfers it to the employee in writing. Such a work is referred to in the Copyright Act as a *work made for hire*. "The rationale for this rule is that the work is produced under the employer's direction and expense; also the employer bears the risks and should be allowed to reap the benefits" (Dible, 1978, p. 130). Your employer, however, would not be entitled to the copyright on a work you authored that was not prepared within the scope of your employment. If you plan to author something from which you hope to profit financially and if you will be doing it wholly or partially "on the job" and/or at your employer's expense, your employer may feel that he or she will be entitled to ownership of the copyright on it. To avoid a misunderstanding when the "work" is completed, it probably would be a good idea before beginning it to request a letter from your employer acknowledging your right to copy-right the work in your name (or if your employer contributes significantly to the creation of it, in both your names).

Why might an author wish to transfer his or her rights to a work to somebody else? The reason in most cases would be that the author expected to profit from doing so. A publisher, for example, may agree to pay the author a royalty on each copy of his work sold in exchange for this transfer of rights. An author can sometimes negotiate a contract that allows him or her to retain the copyright on a work and then only sell (usually through an agent) certain rights to publishers (e.g., translation rights). By negotiating this type of contract the author is in effect transfer-ring ownership of a part of the copyright.

**Reproduction of Copyrighted Materials
and the Doctrine of Fair Use**

The Copyright Act of 1976 places certain restrictions on prohibiting the reproduction of copyrighted materials. On such restriction has been referred to as the *doctrine of fair use.* For an in-depth discussion of this doctrine, see the Copyright Act and Dible (1978).

The doctrine of fair use, which was developed by the courts, "allows copying without permission from, or payment to, the copyright owner where the use is reasonable and not harmful to the rights of the copyright owner" (Dible, 1978, p. 142). Without this doctrine, no use of copyrighted material would be possible without the copyright owner's permission. The idea here is that certain uses of copyrighted materials are not harmful to the rights of the copyright owner and promote the *public welfare.*

What can be copied under this doctrine? The excerpt from Section 107 of the Act, reproduced below, though somewhat vague, provides some general guidelines:

> ... the fair use of a copyrighted work, including such use by reproduction in copies or phonograph records or by other means ... for purposes such as criticism, comment, news reporting, teaching (including multiple copies for classroom use), scholarship, or research, is not an infringement of copyright. In determining whether the use made of a work in any particular case is a fair use the factors to be considered shall include—
>
> (1) the purpose and character of the use, including whether such use is of a commercial nature or is for nonprofit educational purposes;
> (2) the nature of the copyrighted work;
> (3) the amount and substantiality of the portion used in relation to the copyrighted work as a whole; and
> (4) the effect of the use upon the potential market for or value of the copyrighted work.

In addition to these general guidelines for applying the fair use doctrine, specific ones have been developed for several areas. One such area is teaching. These guidelines permit teachers to make *single copies* of copyrighted materials for use in their teaching. They also permit teachers to make *multiple copies* for classroom use if the number of copies does not exceed the number of pupils in the class and the following restrictions are adhered to:

(1) the copies may not be used as a substitute for anthologies, compilations, or collective works;

(2) copies cannot be made of consumable materials such as work books;

(3) the copies cannot be a substitute for purchases, be "directed by higher authority," or be repeated by the same teacher from term to term; and

(4) there is no charge to the student beyond the actual copying cost (Dible, 1978, p. 143).

Notice of Copyright

It is *desirable* that a copyright notice be placed on all works for which copyright protection is desired. On visually perceptible copies, the notice should contain the following three elements:

(1) the symbol c (the letter C in a circle), or the word "Copyright," or the abbreviation "Copr.";

(2) the year of the first publication of the work; and

(3) the name of the owner of the copyright in the work, or an abbreviation by which the name can be recognized, or a generally known designation of the owner (Dible, 1978, pp. 228–229).

However, "subject to certain safeguards for innocent infringers, protection would not be lost by the complete omission of the notice from large numbers of copies or from a whole edition, if registration of the work is made before or within *five years after publication* [italics mine]" (Dible, 1978, p. 165). Hence, immediate, formal application for a copyright is not a prerequisite for placing a copyright notice on a work or for securing copyright protection for it. The mere placement of a copyright notice on a work ordinarily is sufficient to discourage persons from copying it without permission. The formal registration of a copyright, however, does increase the number of types of remedies that its owner can seek from a court.

Deposit and Registration of the Work
for Which Copyright Protection is Sought

The formal copyrighting of a work ordinarily involves (1) depositing two complete copies in the Library of Congress and (2) completing an application for copyright registration and paying the required fee. (For an in-depth description of the application procedure, see Chickering & Hartman, 1987.) Depositing the two copies of the work in the Library of Congress isn't always a prerequisite for securing copyright protection. It would not be one if fewer than five copies of the work have been published or the work is an expensive limited edition with numbered copies for which the requirement to deposit two copies would be burdensome, unfair, or unreasonable (see Section 407C of the 1976 Copyright Act). A slide-tape presentation or a videotape production that a speech-language pathologist or audiologist publishes in a limited edition *may* be exempt from the deposit requirement.

Copyright Infringement and Remedies

Owners of a copyright can seek several types of remedies from a court if the copyright is infringed. They can ask the court to issue an *injunction or restraining order* that will temporarily or permanently prevent or stop infringements. They can ask the court to *impound* all allegedly infringing copies of the work during the time a suit for infringement is pending. They can ask the court to award *compensatory damages* which would offset the profits they lost because of the sale of the infringer's copies. Or they can ask the court to award them *statutory damages,* which are a type of punitive damages (see Chapter 2) that defendants can be required to pay simply because they infringed the plaintiff's copyright. They are referred to as *statutory* damages because they are specified in the statute, or law.

For further information about United States copyright law, see Kozak (1990) and Strong (1990).

PROVISIONS OF U.S. PATENT LAW

The regulations pertaining to U.S. patents, when this section was written, were contained in the 1952 Revision of the Patent Law, which came into effect on January 1, 1953. The law is quite complex and it will not be possible to give an in-depth presentation of it here. The law is reprinted in a pamphlet entitled *Patent Laws,* which is sold by the U.S. Government Printing Office, and it is discussed in Dible (1978).

Subject Matter That Can Be Patented

Practically anything *new and useful* that is made as well as practically any *new process* for making useful things is patentable. The Law states that any person who "invents or discovers any new and useful process, machine, manufacture, or composition of matter, or any new and useful improvements thereof, may obtain a patent." Hence, a speech-language pathologist or audiologist who creates a "new and useful" device for evaluating or treating persons who are communicatively handicapped could apply for and probably obtain a patent for it. An example of such a device would be one intended to augment the communication ability of certain severely communicatively impaired children or adults (Silverman, 1989). A perusal of advertisements in the journal *Asha* and a walk through the commercial exhibit area at an ASHA national convention is one way to become more knowledgeable about the types of devices intended to benefit the communicatively handicapped that can be patented.

The term *useful* as applied to devices on which patents are sought has a specific meaning. According to Dible:

> The term "useful" in this connection refers to the condition that the subject matter has a useful purpose and also includes operativeness, that is, a machine that would not operate to perform the intended purpose would not be called useful.

Hence, when you apply for a patent on a device you are *supposed to* be able to demonstrate that it will perform the function(s) you claim it will perform. I italicized the words "supposed to" in the preceding sentence because U.S. patents have been granted to devices intended to help persons who are communicatively handicapped that don't work. Van Riper (1973), for example, has described a number of such devices with U.S. patents that were intended to cure stuttering.

The term *new* as applied to devices on which patents are sought also has a specific meaning. The Statute states that an "invention" will *not* be regarded as new (and, hence, cannot be patented) if one of the following applies:

(a) The invention was known or used by others in this country, or patented or described in a printed publication in this or a foreign country, before the invention thereof by the applicant for patent, or

(b) The invention was patented or described in a printed publication in this or a foreign country or in public use or on sale in this country more than one year prior to the date of the application for patent in the United States.

In addition, the invention (creation) must be sufficiently different from the most nearly similar thing which has been patented that a *reasonable person* would regard the difference as more than trivial—that is, would regard it as an "invention over the prior art" (Dible, 1978, p. 4).

Suppose that you create (invent) a test or therapy tool that consists of printed matter. Can it be patented? The courts have held that printed matter cannot be patented (Dible, 1978), although it can, of course, be copyrighted. The same probably would be true for tests and therapy tools that consist largely of visual images (i.e., photographs and drawings).

Applying for a Patent

The inventor of a device is the only one who can apply for a patent on it, assuming that he or she is alive and *legally competent* (see Chapter 2). It is a crime for anyone to falsely state that he or she is the inventor of a device and apply for a patent on it. For this reason, any controversy about who invented a device should be resolved before an attempt is made to patent it. Colleagues, for example, might claim that their suggestions contributed significantly to your invention and, therefore, they should share in the financial benefits that you receive from it.

Perhaps the first thing to consider when deciding whether to apply for a patent is whether the market for the device is sufficiently large that you are likely to benefit financially from patenting it. Applying for a patent can be costly in both time and money. People sometimes don't patent inventions because they feel that doing so would be unlikely to yield a reasonable financial return.

If you decide to patent your invention, it may be important for you to be able to document the date on which you first conceived of the idea. This can be done by having persons whom you told about the invention state in writing the date on which they first recall you describing it to them and/or the date on which they first read a description of it. Such documentation can be useful if someone claims to have invented the same thing at an earlier date.

Since an invention must be *new* to be patentable, a necessary step in filing a patent application is demonstrating that no similar device has been patented in the United States or elsewhere. This involves making a systematic search of existing patents. This search ordinarily is made in the Search Room of the Patent and Trademark Office. The inventor may make the search or hire a patent practitioner to make it. If the search does not reveal any similar devices, he or she can prepare and file a patent application.

A patent application has several parts. One is an oath in which the person filing the application declares that he or she is the original, first, and sole inventor of the device for which a patent is sought. The results of the patent search support this declaration. Another part is a detailed description of the invention and a drawing of it. Ordinarily, an inventor retains a patent attorney or a patent agent (i.e., a patent specialist who is not an attorney) to assist in preparing the application and filing it in the Patent and Trademark Office.

After the application is filed it is examined by a Patent and Trademark Office examiner. The examiner decides whether the invention has been properly described and also performs a patent search to verify the inventor's declaration that the invention is new. When the examiner is convinced that the invention is new and useful and that the application has been prepared properly, he or she will recommend that a patent be granted.

Once inventors have been granted a patent they may sell, or assign, the patent to someone who wishes to manufacture and market the invention. They may retain the patent and license its use by one or more manufacturers. Or they may decide to manufacture and market the invention themselves.

Notice of Patent

A notice of patent must be attached to all patented articles. The notice should consist of the word "Patent" and the number of the patent. The patentee (i.e., the one who owns a patent) ordinarily cannot recover damages from an infringer if the appropriate notice was not attached to the patented article in question.

Some articles have the words "patent applied for" or "patent pending" on them. These words merely indicate that a patent has been applied for. The invention is not legally protected from patent infringement until the patent is granted.

Patent Infringement and Remedies

Infringement of a patent is "the unauthorized making, using, or selling of the patented invention within the territory of the United States during the term of the patent" (Dible, 1978, p. 26). The types of remedies that a court can grant for patent infringement are essentially the same as those that were mentioned elsewhere in this chapter for copyright infringement.

Chapter IX

LEGAL ASPECTS OF
ADMINISTRATION AND PRIVATE PRACTICE

The delivery of speech, language, and hearing services to the communicatively handicapped is viewed by the government as a *business*
and as such is subject to the laws that regulate businesses. That a clinical
facility has no prospect of making a profit—which is the case for many
facilities delivering speech, language, and/or hearing services—does not
exclude it from being classified in this manner (Black, 1968, p. 249).
Hence, speech-language pathologists and audiologists are regarded as
operating a business, regardless of whether they are in private practice
or are functioning within an institution such as a hospital or school
system. On this basis they are subject to certain state and federal regulations (e.g., those pertaining to discrimination in employment). Anyone
who administers a unit providing services to the communicatively
handicapped—even a unit employing only one clinician who is also the
administrator—must be aware of these regulations.

Some aspect of business law that have relevance for establishing and
administering a clinical facility will be described in this chapter. I shall
begin by discussing the three types of legal structures (i.e., single
proprietorship, partnership, and corporation) that can be used for orga-
nizing a private practice. Legal aspects of the employer-employee relationship will be considered next, including some types of statutes that
regulate this relationship. Legally and ethically acceptable forms of
advertising will then be indicated. Finally, the types of records that must
be kept for tax and other purposes will be considered.

ORGANIZATIONAL STRUCTURES
FOR PRIVATE PRACTICES

Three basic approaches to business organization have been used by
private practices offering clinical services to the communicatively handi-

capped: individual ownership (or proprietorship), partnership, and incorporation. The advantages and disadvantages of these three organizational forms—particularly as they apply to private practice in speech-language pathology and audiology—will be indicated in this section.

Individual Ownership

Individual ownership (or single proprietorship) is regarded as the least complex of these organizational forms. It is the type that is most likely to be adopted by a speech-language pathologist or audiologist who is beginning a private practice, particularly a part-time one. When this organizational form is used, the business (e.g., a private practice) is owned by a single person. More than half the businesses in this country are individually owned. The owner may employ other persons, including other professionals. An audiologist, for example, may own a hearing aid dealership that employs several other audiologists and a secretary. Two advantages of individual ownership are that the owner is responsible only to himself or herself and reaps the profits if the enterprise is successful. Another possible advantage is that the legal costs of establishing a business using this form tend to be less than when either of the others is used. The main disadvantage of this organizational form is that the owner is entirely responsible for any debts and losses that the business incurs. This would mean, for example, that if a private practice was not successful financially, the owner would have to pay all persons owed money (e.g., employees and the landlord) from personal funds. If these were not sufficient to cover the debts, creditors could ask a court to order that the owner's home and other possessions be sold. Hence, the failure of an individually owned business can lead to the financial ruin of its owner. A person beginning a business—at least partially for this reason—may opt for one of the other organizational forms.

Partnership

Partnership differs from individual ownership in that a business is owned by two or more persons rather than a single person. Any number of persons can enter into a partnership. Those entering into a partnership invest their money or their services or both. An audiologist could begin a hearing aid dealership by investing his or her services and by locating one or more persons who were willing to invest the money needed for the purpose. Or two audiologists could begin a hearing aid dealership by investing both their money and their services. A written agreement, or contract (see Chapter 5), usually is drawn up that specifies the rights and duties of all participants in the partnership. The partners share equally in both the profits and the losses of the business unless the agreement specifies otherwise. If there are losses, the partners are obliged to pay them from their own personal resources. Hence, one advantage of partnership over individual ownership is that the losses (if there are any) are shared—that is, they are not the responsibility of a single person. A partnership agreement may be for a limited or indefinite period of time, depending on the needs of the partners.

Corporation

One disadvantage of both individual ownership and partnership is that any losses incurred by a business have to be paid by its owner or owners (partners) from their own personal resources. Thus, a speech-language pathologist or audiologist who uses one of these organizational forms to establish a private practice not only risks not making a living if the practice is unsuccessful, but also risks having to use personal property to pay its debts.

One advantage of the corporate structure over the other two is that it protects the owner(s) of a business from personal liability if there are losses. [While this is true for large corporations, it may not be true for small ones such as private practices—see Hoops and Sliwoski (1988).] "A corporation obtains its financing by selling stock, or shares of ownership, and the liability of a stockholder in almost all situations is limited to the cost of the stock for which he subscribes" (You and the Law, *1977, p. 509*).

The reason for the owners and officers of a corporation having limited personal liability is that a corporation is classified by the courts as a *person* —i.e., an independent entity. A corporation can buy and sell property in its own name, and it can commit crimes and torts and be tried and punished for them. Businesses established as single proprietorships or partnerships are not regarded by the courts as independent entities, but as extensions of their owners. Hence, the property of a single proprietorship or partnership is regarded by the courts as belonging to its owner or owners. Thus, the initiating of a court action against a single proprietorship or partnership involves suing its owner or owners.

A corporation acquires its status as an independent legal entity on the basis of how it is formed. "A corporation is a group of people who obtain a charter from the state government that grants them, as a unit, some of the legal rights, powers, and abilities of a human being for conducting any lawful activities" (*You and the Law,* 1977, p. 508). The state endows it with perpetual existence. A corporation continues to exist even after all the persons responsible for obtaining its charter either die or sell their interest in it. It does not cease to exist until it is dissolved by the appropriate legal procedure.

A charter for a corporation is granted by a state government rather than the federal government. Ordinarily, a charter is sought from the state in which the owners of the corporation live and in which the corporation will transact a significant proportion of its business. Sometimes, however, the charter is sought from a state other than the one in which the owners live. The state from which they are most likely to seek a charter in such instances is *Delaware.* This is because the tax and other laws applicable to corporations in Delaware are viewed as being more favorable than those of other states (Nicholas, 1977). While a corporation can function in a state other the one in which it was chartered, in such a state it probably would be viewed as a "foreign" corporation and for this reason may be treated differently from a corporation that was chartered in that state.

An organization does not have to be large to incorporate. It is theoretically possible in some states (e.g., Delaware) for a single individual to apply for and obtain a charter for a corporation. A private practice in speech-language pathology and audiology probably could be incorporated in such a state.

The main *disadvantages* of the corporate structure are (1) it tends to be more expensive to establish (e.g., with respect to legal fees) than the partnership or single proprietorship and (2) the amount of tax paid on income is likely to be higher than on individual income. Prior to the passage of the Tax Reform Act of 1986, it often was possible to "spread the income stream over two sets of marginal tax brackets and pay a reduced amount of income taxes" (Hoops & Silwoski, 1988, p. 44). An accountant can advise you about whether in your particular situation there would be any tax or other financial advantage to incorporating.

LEGAL ASPECTS OF THE
EMPLOYER–EMPLOYEE RELATIONSHIP

Most speech-language pathologists and audiologists function as employees, employers, or both. If you are receiving a salary for your services, you would ordinarily be regarded as an employee. If you hire people and they are paid a salary for their services by you or your institution, you would ordinarily be regarded as an employer. And if you are both receiving a salary and involved in the hiring of other persons, you ordinarily would be looked upon as functioning in both roles. Hence, a person functioning as the administrator (part- or full-time) of speech, language, and/or hearing services in an institution such as a public school or hospital probably would be functioning as an employer as well as an employee and, consequently, would have to be aware of legal aspects of the employer role.

Master-Servant, Principal-Agent, and Employer-Independent-Contractor Relationships

The specific legal responsibilities of an employer to an employee and of an employee to an employer depend on whether their relationship would be most likely to be viewed by the courts as that of a *master to a servant* or a *principal to an agent*, or an *employer to an independent contractor.* The legal responsibilities of an employer to an employee in a specific situation are determined by whether in that situation the employer is functioning as a "master," a "principal," or an "employer." The relationship with a particular employee in some situations may be that of a master to a servant; in others it may be that of a principal to an agent or an employer to an independent contractor. The terms *master* and *servant* as used in this context do not have their usual meanings; their meanings here are more metaphorical than literal.

One of the main differences among these three types of relationships is the amount of responsibility that the employer assumes for the activities of the employee. The employer assumes more responsibility for them in the master-servant relationship than in the principal-agent one. He or she assumes least responsibility for these activities in the employer-independent-contractor relationship.

What are the characteristics of a *master-servant relationship?* According to Black:

> The relationship of master and servant exists where one person, for pay or other valuable consideration [e.g., "hours" toward satisfying a clinical practicum requirement] enters into the service of another and devotes to him his personal labor for an agreed period . . . It usually contemplates employer's right to *prescribe* [italics mine] end and direct means and method of doing work (1968, p. 1127).

Hence, in this type of relationship the employer (or someone whom the employer has authorized to act in his or her behalf) prescribes not only *what* the employee is to do, but *how* he or she is to do it. A master-servant relationship would exist between a speech-language pathologist and a paraprofessional communication aide if the speech-language pathologist prescribes not only the type of therapy the paraprofessional is to administer but how it is to be administered. It also would tend to exist between a speech-language pathologist or audiologist functioning as a practicum supervisor and a student clinician.

Because an employee in a master-servant relationship theoretically is following orders, the person giving the orders (e.g., the person prescribing therapy) is legally responsible for any damage done to person or property by the employee which resulted from the orders being carried out. This is referred to as *vicarious liability* because the person who does the "deed" is not the one who has to assume responsibility for it (Woody, 1986). Physicians have traditionally had relationships of this type with nurses, physical therapists, occupational therapists, and other health professionals who deliver services that they prescribe. Some relatively recent court decisions, however, have held such persons partially responsible for damage done to patients as a consequence of a prescription being carried out. Health professionals are particularly likely to be expected to share responsibility for such damage if they are aware that a prescribed treatment they are administering to a patient is likely to be harmful. Because speech-language pathologists and audiologists ordinarily do not work under a physician's prescription, they are not exempted from legal responsibility for any damage that they do to clients.

What are the characteristics of a *principal-agent relationship?* According to Black, an agent is

> one who deals not only with things, as does a servant, but with persons, *using his own discretion as to means* [italics mine], and frequently establishes contractual relations between his principal and third persons (1968, pp. 85–86).

An "agent," therefore, differs from a "servant" in the following two ways: First, an agent ordinarily is not told specifically how to carry out assigned duties, but is permitted to use "his own discretion as to means." For example, a speech-language pathologist employed by a school system who is functioning in this role would be told to provide clinical services to children at a particular school, but the particular children he or she served and how he or she served them would be left to his or her own discretion.

A second way in which an agent differs from a servant is that agents can *establish contractual relations* between their employer (i.e., principal) and third persons. For example, a public-school speech-language pathologist would be establishing a contractual relationship between her employer and a particular test publisher (third person) when she ordered a diagnostic test from that publisher for use in her school—that is, she would be obligating her employer to pay for the test.

Speech-language pathologists and audiologists who are employed by schools, hospitals, or other institutions ordinarily function as agents. Consequently, they have to assume some legal responsibility for any damage they do to their clients. They probably would not have to assume the full responsibility if they committed a tort because a court would be likely to view the employer (principal) as tacitly certifying their professionalism and competence by employing them. Hence, an employer probably would have to assume some of responsibility for any damage that a clinician did to a client.

What are the characteristics of an *employer-independent-contractor relationship?* According to Black, an independent contractor is

> one who, exercising an independent employment, contracts to do a piece of work according to his own methods and without being subject to the control of his employer except as to the results of the work (1968, p. 911).

Hence, "independent contractors" differ from "agents" and "servants" in several ways. First, they are self-employed. They contract with their employers to do a particular piece of work. An audiologist, for example, might contract with an industrial firm to screen its employees for noise-induced hearing loss for an agreed-upon fee per employee. The audiologist would not be an employee of the firm. He or she would be a self-employed professional who was paid a fee to perform "a piece of work" (i.e., a hearing screening). After the hearing tests were administered and the results reported, his or her relationship with the firm would end.

A second way that independent contractors differ from agents and servants (particularly the latter) is that their employers ordinarily do not specify how the work is to be performed. They specify the desired results in the contract and ordinarily leave the means to the discretion of the independent contractor. The audiologist in our previous example to fulfill the contract would have to report the status of each employee's hearing to the firm. He or she could use any audiometric testing procedure that would be expected to yield data possessing adequate levels of validity and reliability.

A third way that independent contractors differ from agents and servants is that they have to assume full responsibility for any damage that they do. Speech-language pathologists and audiologists in private practice are independent contractors. As such, they have to assume full responsibility for any harm they bring about. They would be wise, therefore, to purchase professional liability insurance. Information about companies that sell such insurance can be obtained from the American Speech-Language-Hearing Association.

Thus far, we have considered the employer-employee relationship primarily from the perspective of the employee. When we consider the role of the employee as a servant, agent, or independent contractor from an *employer's perspective,* one of the main concerns is the employer's responsibility for his or her employees' work-related torts and broken (breached) contracts. The concept that one person can be held responsible for another person's torts and broken contracts is referred to in the legal literature as the doctrine of *respondeat superior.* "The fundamental rule generally recognized is that the doctrine of *respondeat superior* is applicable to the relation of master and servant or of principal and agent, but not to that of employer and independent contractor" (from court opinion in *Miller v. Metropolitan Live Insurance Company, 134 Ohio St. 289*). Hence, employers can protect themselves from responsibility for the work-related torts and broken contracts of their employees by utilizing independent contractors. A nursing home, for example, probably could protect itself from tort litigation associated with the delivery of speech, language, and hearing services by contracting with a private practitioner for their delivery.

Government Regulation of the Employer-Employee Relationship

Many aspects of the employer-employee relationship are regulated directly or indirectly by either the state and federal government. These include the following: (1) factors to consider when deciding whether to hire, fire, or promote someone; (2) the nature of the physical work environment; (3) the manner in which employer-employee disputes are settled; and (4) the compensation of employees for their services. Some implications of each are indicated in the following paragraphs.

An employer ordinarily is not permitted to hire, fire, or promote employees strictly on the basis of whether or not he or she likes them. A number of laws prohibit discrimination in hiring and promotion on the basis of extraneous (to the requirements of the job) employee characteristics such as age, gender, race, religion, sexual preference and/or possession of a disability. Some regulations go one step further. They require preference to be given in hiring and promotion to persons against whom society has discriminated in the past. This is referred to as *affirmative action.*

The government also regulates to some extent the conditions under which work is performed. The main thrust of government regulation in this area appears to be the minimizing of hazards to workers' health. One federal administrative agency that is quite involved with this area is the Occupational Safety and Health Administration (OSHA). An example of an aspect of the work environment that OSHA has attempted to regulate is ambient noise level.

The government has also made some attempt to regulate how disputes between employers and employees are resolved. Persons associated with government agencies have been instrumental in arbitrating such disputes. The government is unlikely to do so, however, unless a dispute is viewed as seriously threatening the public interest.

Many government regulations deal with how employees are to be compensated for their services. They deal with such matters as the minimum wage that can be offered an employee, employers' and employees' contributions to employees' social security accounts, and the percentages of wages that must be withheld for state and federal income taxes.

ADVERTISING

Professionals advertise to make potential consumers aware of their services. Speech-language pathologists and audiologists traditionally have adhered to the ethical restrictions on advertising adopted by other independent health professionals, such as physicians and dentists. Prior to the 1970s, direct advertising of clinical services was restricted to such activities as listing oneself in the appropriate section of the "yellow pages" of the telephone book and placing a "dignified" announcement in local newspapers when beginning a private practice. Physicians and other health professionals are no longer restricted to these. Consequently, speech-language pathologists and audiologists are not either. Support for this conclusion is provided by the following statement from the 1991 ASHA Ethical Code:

> Individuals should announce services in a manner consonant with highest professional standards in the community.

Ethical restrictions on the advertising of clinical services offered by health professionals were relaxed somewhat during the late 1970s, in part, because of a 1978 Supreme Court decision (*United States v. National Society of Professional Engineers*) in which "the Court found that it was illegal for any professional society to hold its members to an ethical code which had the effect of limiting competition among its members" (Del Polito, 1979, p. 924). An ethical code that placed restraints on advertising could be interpreted as having the effect of limiting competition.

RECORD KEEPING FOR
TAX AND OTHER BUSINESS PURPOSES

A clinical facility is classified as a business, and hence is required to keep some of the types of records that other businesses do. The specific types that must be kept are determined, in part, by whether the facility is organized as a single proprietorship, a partnership, or a cooperation and whether it is intended to be a for-profit or a non-profit entity. It is important before opening a clinical facility (e.g., a private practice) to have an accountant develop a record-keeping system that will yield the information required for meeting municipal, state, and federal statutes and regulations concerned with taxes and other regulated aspects of business management.

ADDENDUM

Further information about business aspects of clinical practice in speech-language pathology and audiology can be obtained from the American Speech-Language-Hearing Association and the American Academy of Private Practice in Speech-Language Pathology and Audiology. This aspect of clinical practice is one of the main ones with which the Academy is concerned. The following books provide helpful information about business aspects of clinical practice: *Private practice in Communication Disorders,* by Wood (1986); *Private Practice in Audiology and Speech Pathology,* edited by Battin and Fox (1978); *Prospering in Private Practice,* edited by Butler (1986); and *Speech and Language Procedure Manual,* by Lehrhoff and Koroshec (no date).

Chapter X

LEGAL AND ETHICAL
CONSIDERATIONS IN CLINICAL RESEARCH

Almost all of the research conducted by speech-language pathologists and audiologists involves the use of human subjects. Persons who have participated in such research have been harmed by the failure of investigators to foresee possible undesirable effects of their experimental procedures on them (see Metz & Folkins, 1985; Silverman, 1988). There has been considerable interest since the Nuremberg trials, which were conducted after World War II for "crimes against humanity" committed by persons in Germany associated with the Third Reich (see Hoedeman, 1991; International Auschwitz Committee, 1986), and the breaking of the story in 1972 about a study of the long term effects of syphilis that was conducted by the United States Public Health Service for 40 years in which many poor black men who had the disease were denied treatment for it (Jones, 1981) in the mental and physical welfare of persons who serve as subjects in research studies. This interest has resulted in the creation of regulations on both national and international levels (see Appendix B) that are intended to protect the rights of such persons. It also has stimulated considerable discussion about ethical aspects of how human subjects are used in research (see Freund, 1970; Levine, 1986; Reece & Siegal, 1986; Schuler, 1982; Veatch, 1987).

A number of legal and ethical considerations in clinical research are discussed in this chapter. Much of this discussion is also applicable to other kinds of research in which human subjects are used.

NEED FOR PROTECTING RESEARCH SUBJECTS

Persons who volunteer to serve as subjects are likely to assume that they will be *protected by the experimenter* from being harmed in any way. They would be particularly likely to make this assumption if they are volunteering to participate in an experiment from which they could not

expect to benefit personally. Subjects can benefit personally by participating in an experiment in several ways, such as gaining knowledge,
improving physical and/or mental health, or being paid (Macklin, 1989).
They also would be particularly likely to make it if the research was
being conducted under the auspices of a respected institution (such as a
university or hospital).

While subjects may assume that there is no possibility of their being
harmed by participating in an experiment, such an assumption would
not be valid. It is impossible to design an experiment that is entirely
risk-free. One of the most difficult components of the ethical review of
research proposals by institutional review boards (IRBs) is assessing
potential risks of harm to research participants (Meslin, 1990; Thompson,
1990).

Although it would be unrealistic for subjects to assume that their
participation in an experiment is entirely risk-free, it would not be
unreasonable for them to assume that their risk of being harmed is
almost nonexistent if they are not informed to the contrary (Greenwald,
Ryan, & Mulvihill, 1982). Hence, an experimenter who exposed subjects
to more than extremely minimal risks of harm *without first informing them*
about these risks would probably be viewed as behaving irresponsibly.
The subjects, if they were harmed, could sue both the experimenter and
the institution under whose auspices the research was conducted for
negligence and/or some other tort (possibly *battery*) with a reasonable
expectation of winning (Feuer, 1990). This is one of the reasons why
institutions have review boards (IRBs) to evaluate research proposals.
(For information about the functioning of these boards see Greenwald,
Ryan, & Mulvihill (1982) and the newsletter *IRB: A Review of Human
Subjects Research.*)

It is important that the actual risk of harm to a subject be consistent
with the subject's assumption regarding the nature of this risk. How can
one insure that this will be the case? Several approaches can be used to
insure that a subject's *consent* to participate in an experiment is *informed.*
One would be to rely on the *experimenter* both to minimize risks to
subjects and to inform them voluntarily about the risks remaining.
While this would be the simplest (and probably the most common)
approach, it has several limitations. Perhaps its main limitation is that
the goals of collecting desired data and of protecting the persons from
whom these data are being collected may not be compatible. Ordinarily
an experimenter's primary objective is to gather the data needed to

answer specific questions or to test specific hypotheses. While few experimenters would knowingly expose their subjects to highly danger- ous experimental conditions without informing them about the risks, they might be tempted to be less forthright when there are potential risks associated with them that have not been demonstrated unequivocally to exist. Experimenters may hesitate to inform potential subjects about such risks because it could discourage enough of them from volunteering to make it impossible for the study to be undertaken or completed.

A second approach that can be used for insuring that a subject's consent to participate is informed and that potential risks have been minimized and are within acceptable limits is to require the designs of all research studies that wish to use institutional clients as subjects to be scrutinized by an *institutional research board*. The mission of this board would be to identify potential risks and to determine both whether they are within acceptable limits and whether subjects will be fully informed about them (Metz & Folkins, 1985). This approach has been adopted by many institutions, including school systems, universities, and hospitals. Requiring such a board to approve the design for a study can protect subjects in several ways. First, it would probably motivate the experimenter to design the study so as to minimize the risks to subjects and thus maximize the odds of the proposal's being approved by the board. Also, the experimenter would hesitate to propose a study that would expose subjects to unacceptably high risks of harm because doing so could damage his or her professional reputation. Second, such a board pro- vides a mechanism for monitoring the degree to which subjects are informed about potential hazards and hence the degree to which their consent constitutes *informed consent*. Institutional research boards may require experimenters to submit to them copies of the consent forms that subjects will be asked to sign. The board would then decide whether the presentation of possible hazards on them is sufficiently complete and accurate for a subject's consent to constitute fully informed consent. If a subject is not fully informed about potential hazards before signing a consent form, his or her consent probably would not be recognized by a court (Greenwald, Ryan, & Mulvihill, 1982). The concept of informed consent is dealt with in-depth elsewhere in this chapter.

While the second approach (using institutional review boards) tends to be superior to the first (relying solely on the experimenter) for protecting the rights of subjects, it is not perfect. One of its limitations is that board members may not be sufficiently familiar with the topic to assess either its scientific worthyness or the adequacy of the methodology to achieve its purpose and protect subjects from harm. "It is well established that for research involving human beings to be ethical it must be scientifically worthy" (Freedman, 1987, p. 7). It is also well established that for such research to be ethical, the methodology being proposed must be such that it is likely to yield the information needed to achieve its purpose (McLarty, 1987) while minimizing the risk of harm to subjects.

INFORMED CONSENT AS A VEHICLE FOR PROTECTING INVESTIGATORS AND INSTITUTIONS

Clinical research in the previous section was viewed from the perspective of the need for protecting the rights of research subjects. In this section it will be viewed from a different perspective—that of the need for protecting the rights of investigators and the institutions under whose auspices they are doing their research. If our legal system did not protect these rights, little (if any) clinical research would be undertaken, which would have an obvious detrimental impact on the health of persons in our society.

Securing subjects' *informed consent* to participate in a study can provide both the investigator(s) and the institution under whose auspices the research is being conducted with some protection against litigation arising from allegations that they were physically or mentally harmed by doing so (Greenwald, Ryan, & Mulvihill, 1982). If they were aware of a particular risk before consenting to participate in the study and if they were harmed in a manner predictable from this risk, they would be unlikely to be successful if they sued either the investigator or the institution.

One of the main types of litigation against which a subject's informed consent to participate in a study can provide some protection is *battery*. According to Fried:

The central concept of battery is the offense to personal dignity that occurs when another impinges on one's bodily integrity without full and valid consent. A punch in the stomach or being doused with a pail of water are classic examples. It is not necessary to show that one has been physically injured, much less that one has suffered financial loss. The injury is to dignity. That being the case, law suits have been brought and won against doctors who performed needed and successful operations, but without consent of their patients (1974, p. 15).

Hence, experimenting on people without their "full and valid consent" can result in litigation for battery even if they were not physically injured and even if they did not suffer financial loss. Such litigation also can result for subjecting clients to *therapy programs* without their "full and valid consent." For further information about battery and other torts for which an investigator can be sued, see Chapter 6.

The requirement that must be satisfied to justify intentionally invading another's bodily integrity is securing his or her *free and informed* consent to do so. According to Fried:

> To be effective the consent must be to the particular contact with the person in question, and if procured by "fraud or mistake as to the essential character" of the conduct it is invalid.... And it is not just active fraud or concealment which destroys consent. The doctor [or experimenter] who obtains consent has the duty to give the facts the patient [or subject] needs to make an informed choice.... He must tell the patient [or subject] about the benefits and risks of the treatment [or experimental condition(s)], and how likely they are. And some courts have said that the patient must also be told about the hazards and advantages of alternative forms of treatment (1974, pp. 19–20).

Hence, for consent to participate in an experiment to be regarded by a court as having been *free and informed*, the experimenter would have to be able to prove that subjects were not coerced into giving it and that they had been fully informed (i.e., had not been deceived) about the risks involved before they gave it (Cupples & Gochnauer, 1985).

Under some circumstances a subject's free and informed consent to participate in a study *may* not be essential. One such circumstance would be when the subject is a *child*, particularly a very young child who would be unable to understand the study and hence would be incapable of giving informed consent. Consent in such a circumstance would have to be obtained from the child's legal guardian, who in most instances would be a parent. However, a guardian's ability to consent to a child's serving as a research subject is limited: "The tendency of the law has been to limit what may be done to children and incompetents just because they are unable to give effective consent. And those who act for them are strictly charged to act only in the manifest interests of these persons. They may not, for instance, volunteer them for experimentation which will *not directly* [italics mine] benefit them" (Fried, 1974, p. 23). The message here appears to be that securing a guardian's consent for his or her child to serve as a subject may not be adequate to protect against litigation either the experimenter or the institution under whose auspices the research is being conducted.

A subject's free and informed consent also may not be essential if he or she is an adult whom the court would classify as *incompetent.* Adults are likely to be classified as incompetent if they are thought to be unable to make rational decisions regarding their own welfare. Persons diagnosed as psychotic or severely mentally retarded are likely to be classified as incompetent. Persons who are *severely communicatively handicapped* (e.g., global aphasics) also may be classified as incompetent. A court-appointed guardian could consent to such a person's serving as a subject: The restrictions on the guardian's ability to do so are the same as were given for guardians of children.

A subject can *withdraw* consent to participate in a study at any time, even if the subject promised when giving consent not to withdraw it (Greenwald, Ryan, & Mulvihill, 1982). Some persons argue, however, that investigators should be allowed to impose some limits on a subject's right to do so (Newton, 1982). The National Institute of Health policy statement on the protection of human subjects has not only mandates that subjects be allowed to withdraw consent at any time but requires that subjects *be informed* that they have this right.

For further information about informed consent for research subjects, see Fletcher, Dommel, Jr., & Cowell (1985), Greenwald, Ryan, & Mulvihill (1982), Grinnell (1990), Newton (1982), Levine (1983), Taub (1986), and Weithorn (1983).

LEGAL-ETHICAL IMPLICATIONS OF THE THERAPEUTIC-NONTHERAPEUTIC CONTINUUM IN CLINICAL RESEARCH

The legal doctrines that apply to a particular clinical study are determined in part by whether the experimental conditions administered to subjects are intended to be therapeutic to them. Some studies are *entirely therapeutic* in their intent. An example would be a study of the impacts of a particular intervention program that the clinician would have used it even if the research was not being done.

At the other end of the continuum would be studies in which the investigator had *no therapeutic intent*. The subjects in such studies would be unlikely to benefit personally from participating in them. They may, however, be providing data that could contribute to improving therapy programs for others with similar communicative disorders at some future date. An example would be an investigation by an audiologist of the responses of persons having a particular type of lesion in the auditory system to a particular type of auditory test. The audiologist's intent is to use their responses to the test stimuli to refine the test rather than to benefit them directly.

There are clinical studies that fall on the continuum between these extremes. In these studies some of the experimental conditions have a therapeutic intent and others do not. Or the experimental conditions are intended to be therapeutic for some subjects but not for others. An example of the first would be a study in which clients are given one or more diagnostic tests in addition to those they would ordinarily be given for clinical purposes. Those that ordinarily would be administered for clinical purposes constitute experimental conditions having a therapeutic intent; the others constitute experimental conditions that are not intended to be therapeutic.

An example of a clinical study in which the experimental conditions are intended to be therapeutic for some subjects but not for others would be a study in which subjects are *randomly assigned* to one of two treatment groups. The subjects assigned to the first group (the experimental group) would be administered a treatment (experimental condition) that was intended to be therapeutic and hence could directly benefit them. Those assigned to the second group (the control group) either would be administered no treatment or would be administered a treatment that the experimenter did not expect to be as successful as the one administered to subjects in the first group. Thus, the subjects in the first group would be expected to benefit directly, and those in the second group either would not be expected to benefit directly or would not be expected to benefit to the same extent as those in the first group.

Nontherapeutic Clinical Research.

While the persons who function as subjects in nontherapeutic clinical research may receive a small sum of money and/or personal satisfaction for doing so, they are unlikely to benefit directly in any substantial way from the experience. And by participating in the research they are risking their mental and/or physical health. In some types of research the risks to their health would be almost nonexistent; in others the risks would be substantial.

It has been argued (Fried, 1974) that there are no special legal doctrines that apply to nontherapeutic clinical research and that those that do apply (particularly with regard to the need for disclosing potential hazards) are the same as those that apply to the selling of products:

> *In general, the law imposes a strict duty of disclosure, wherever an individual with a great deal to lose is exposed to a risk or is asked to relinquish rights by someone with considerably greater knowledge* [italics mine]. And this is true, whether the relation is one of buyer and seller or involves some public interest. Persons selling cosmetics, automobiles, or pharmaceuticals are required to make full disclosure of all the hazards involved in the products they sell. . . . There is no reason why the case should be any different where a researcher asks an experimental subject to risk his health (Fried, 1974, p. 27).

Since experimenters would ordinarily have considerably greater knowledge of the potential risks associated with the methodology being used than would their subjects and since their subjects are risking their health by participating in the experiment, experimenters are obliged to make a full disclosure of potential hazards to subjects when seeking their consent to participate. It could be argued that the failure of the experimenter to do so would be more damaging with this type of research if a subject sued for battery that it would be with research having a therapeutic intent.

While it is almost always desirable to be able to document a subject's informed consent to participate in research, there are some types of nontherapeutic studies for which failure to do so ordinarily would result in minimal risks to either investigators or the institutions under whose auspices their research is being conducted. These are studies that involve only slight or remote risks of harm to subjects. The U.S. Department of Health and Human Services, for example, in its *Final Regulations Amending Basic HHS Policy for the Protection of Human Research Subjects* (*Federal Register*, January 26, 1981) classified the following types of research as having no, slight, or only remote risks of harm to subjects:

1. Research conducted in established or commonly accepted educational settings, involving normal educational practices, such as (i) research on regular and special education instructional strategies, or (ii) research on the effectiveness of or the comparison

among instructional techniques, curricula, or classroom management methods.

2. Research involving the use of educational tests (cognitive, diagnostic, aptitude, achievement), if information taken from these sources are recorded in such a manner that subjects cannot be identified, directly or through identifiers linked to the subjects.

3. Research involving survey or interview procedures, except where all of the following conditions exist: (i) responses are recorded in such a manner that the human subjects can be identified, directly or through identifiers linked to the subjects, (ii) the subject's responses, if they became known outside the research, could reasonably place the subject at risk of criminal or civil liability or be damaging to the subject's financial standing or employability, and (iii) the research deals with sensitive aspects of the subject's own behavior, such as illegal conduct, drug use, sexual behavior, or the use of alcohol. . . .

   Research involving the observation (including the observation by participants) of public behavior, except where all of the following conditions exist: (i) observations are recorded in such a manner that the human subjects can be identified, directly or through identifiers linked to the subjects, (ii) the observations recorded about the individual, if they become known outside the research, could reasonably place the subject at risk of criminal or civil liability or be damaging to the subject's financial standing or employability, and (iii) the research deals with sensitive aspects of the subject's own behavior such as illegal conduct, drug use, sexual behavior, or use of alcohol.

4. Research involving the collection or study of existing data, documents, pathological specimens, or diagnostic specimens, if these sources are publicly available or if the information is recorded by the investigator in such a manner that subjects cannot be identified, directly or through identifiers linked to the subjects (*Federal Register*, January 26, 1981, pp. 8371–8372).

How would a person be compensated for harm resulting from his or her participation (as a subject) in a nontherapeutic research study? Such a person probably would have to initiate some type of litigation against the investigator and/or the institution under whose auspices the research was being conducted. A number of authorities on legal-ethical implications of using human subjects in research (e.g., Fried, 1974; Ladimer,

1970) have stated that investigators and their institutions have a moral obligation to voluntarily compensate subjects harmed in nontherapeutic research. Perhaps a special liability insurance could be carried by investigators or their institutions for this purpose.

For further information about legal-ethical aspects of nontherapeutic research, see Freund (1970), Fried, (1974), Greenwald, Ryan, and Mulvihill (1982), Levine (1983), Metz and Folkins (1985) and the publications of the Office for Protection from Research Risks, National Institutes of Health, Bethesda, Maryland 20205.

Therapeutic Clinical Research

Speech-language pathologists, audiologists, and other clinicians legally are justified only in using accepted therapies unless their clients specifically consent to the use of an experimental therapy. An *accepted therapy*, in this context, is a treatment program that at least some of one's professional peers would regard as appropriate for the particular condition being treated. If a speech-language pathologist treated a stutterer with a therapy program that at least some authorities on stuttering would regard as appropriate, this program would be likely to be classified as *accepted* therapy by the courts. It would not be necessary that all authorities on stuttering regard it as appropriate. The courts recognize that there are often different "schools of thought" on the appropriate therapy for a condition and, hence, they will classify as accepted almost any therapy advocated by a recognized authority.

So long as the therapy program being used in the research is one that would be classified by the courts as accepted, the legal-ethical considerations (e.g., informed consent) would be essentially the same as for *clinical treatment.*

The further away an experimental therapy program lies from the standard and the accepted, the more acute the need for subjects to be fully informed about risks and *alternative treatment programs*, and the greater the need for the investigator to be able to document the subjects' free and informed consent to participate in research. The investigator's obligation to inform subjects about alternative treatment programs ordinarily does not extend to other alternative programs (Fried, 1974). The information presented about the experimental program should include a statement summarizing research findings and professional opinion relevant to its efficacy.

A situation that may pose a legal-ethical dilemma for an investigator is one in which there are alternative treatment programs that are regarded by other professionals as *effective* for treating the condition the experimental program is intended to treat. Full disclosure requires that the subjects be informed about these alternatives. However, informing potential subjects about such alternatives may cause them to refuse to participate in the experimental program. An investigator may be tempted, therefore, to make a less than full disclosure about alternative treatment programs in order to insure having an adequate number of subjects for the research. While doing so may increase the probability of having an adequate number of subjects for the research, it also could invalidate the subjects' consent to participate in the research, leaving the investigator vulnerable to several types of litigation, including battery. An investigator when confronted with this situation would be wise to make a full disclosure, including a statement summarizing research and professional opinion relevant to why the experimental therapy *may* be superior to existing accepted alternative treatment programs. An investigator should be able to develop such a statement—otherwise, one could reasonably question whether it would be *ethical* to expose subjects to an experimental treatment program that there is no reason to believe is superior to existing accepted ones. Institutional research boards have a responsibility to determine whether proposed experimental treatment programs have a reasonable chance of satisfying a *real need.*

For further information about therapeutic clinical research issues see Freedman (1990) and Grinnell (1990).

Mixed Therapeutic and Nontherapeutic Clinical Research.

The type of clinical research that tends to have the greatest legal-ethical perplexities associated with it is that which has both therapeutic and nontherapeutic aspects. A speech-language pathologist or audiologist, for example, who was engaged in therapy outcome research would indeed by attempting to ameliorate the client's communicative disorder (which would be the *therapeutic aspect*). The intervention strategy chosen, however, would not be selected *solely* from the perspective of the client's needs. Therapy would be administered in the context of a research program that was intended either to test new procedures or to compare the efficacy of various established procedures (which would be the *nontherapeutic aspect.*) Hence, the treatment that a client received would be dictated, at least partially, by the requirements of the research design. In a study of the relative efficacy of two established procedures, the one the client is administered is likely to be determined by a table of random numbers. And in a study of the efficacy of a new procedure (experimental therapy), the decision whether a particular subject would be given it would be partially a function of the investigator's need for subjects with particular *demographic characteristics* (e.g., age and sex) to meet the requirements of the research design.

If the treatment dictated by a research design is the one that a client would have received anyway, then the presence of a research design ordinarily would not create any special legal-ethical problems. However, if the treatment dictated by a research design is *not* the one that a client ordinarily would have received, then the presence of a research design could indicate legal-ethical problems.

In clinical research having both therapeutic and nontherapeutic aspects there obviously is a legal obligation to make a full disclosure of *possible benefits and hazards.* This would be necessary even if the therapy that the clients were receiving was not part of a research project. Would it also be necessary to disclose (1) that at least some of the therapy they will be receiving *is part of a research project* and (2) the *nature* of the research project and the experimental design? A speech-language pathologist who was planning to describe the therapy program used with a client in an individual case study in an article published in a professional journal would have to answer that question. Would the client's consent be needed to publish the case study? If it were *impossible* for anyone to recognize the client from the information included in the case study, the answer to this question probably would be *no.* A client may be recognizable not only from a name or initials but also from specific information about his or her life history, such as the names of schools attended. An investigator would be wise, therefore, to carefully examine the life history data on subjects of case studies and to delete any nonessential information that would make them recognizable. Of course, the client (or the client's guardian) in some instances would be very willing to have a description of the therapy received published, particularly if (1) the client felt treatment was successful and/or (2) the client was convinced that the information presented could help in the treatment of others with similar conditions.

While clinicians who do not disclose to a client that the therapy is part of a research project or do not describe the *impact* that being part of a research project will have on the therapy the client will be receiving may be relatively safe legally, they may find themselves vulnerable from a *public relations* perspective. Most clients, for example, probably would feel that they had been deceived if they discovered they received the therapy program they did because they were randomly assigned to a particular treatment group. Such a discovery would be likely to adversely affect their relationship with their clinician if they are still in therapy. And the disclosure of such a discovery in the media could severely damage the reputation both of the investigator and the institution under whose auspices the research was conducted. The general public would tend to regard the random assignment of subjects to treatment groups without their knowledge as irresponsible, even if the therapy subjects received had been successful.

DOCUMENTING A PERSON'S INFORMED CONSENT TO SERVE AS A RESEARCH SUBJECT

An outline of a form for documenting a person's informed consent to serve as a subject in a research project is presented in Figure 10.1. This outline includes the information that ordinarily is necessary for explaining to potential subjects (1) the purpose and value of the study, (2) what they will be asked to do and what will be done to them, and (3) the possible benefits and risks to them. It also provides a means for documenting that subjects were informed that they may withdraw their consent at any time and that they have consented to having information about them published (if they cannot be recognized). In addition, it provides documentation that their consent was given freely (that it was not coerced or forced). Paragraph *g* in Figure 10.1 would be included only if provision had been made for compensating subjects for injuries that they receive (e.g., if the investigator or the institution had liability insurance that covered such injuries). Note that subjects' signatures should be witnessed. Obviously, if the information presented in the form was inaccurate or incomplete, a subject's signature on it might not constitute *informed* consent. Whether it would constitute informed consent would depend on how essential the inaccurate or incomplete information was for alerting subjects to potential risks.

RESPONSIBLE INVESTIGATOR:

TITLE OF PROTOCOL:

TITLE OF CONSENT FORM *(if different from protocol):*

I have been asked to participate in a research study that is investigating *(describe purpose of study).* In participating in this study I agree to *(describe briefly and in lay terms procedures to which subject is consenting).*

I understand that

a) The possible risks of this procedure include *(list known risks or side effects; if none, so state).* Alternative treatments include *(list alternative treatments and briefly describe advantages and disadvantages of each; if none, so state).*

b) The possible benefits of this study to me are *(enumerate; if none, so state).*

c) Any questions I have concerning my participation in this study will be answered by *(list names and degrees of people who will be available to answer questions).*

d) I may withdraw from the study at any time without prejudice.

e) The results of this study may be published, but my name or identity will not be revealed and my records will remain confidential unless disclosure of my identity is required by law.

f) My consent is given voluntarily without being coerced or forced.

g) In the event of physical injury resulting from the study, medical care and treatment will be available at this institution.

For eligible veterans, compensation (damages) may be payable under 38USC 351 or, in some circumstances, under the Federal Tort claims Act.

For non-eligible veterans and non-veterans, compensation would be limited to situations where negligence occurred and would be controlled by the provisions of the Federal Tort Claims Act.

For clarification of these laws, contact the District Counsel (213) 824-7379.

DATE _____

PATIENT OR RESPONSIBLE PARTY _____

PATIENT'S SOCIAL SECURITY NUMBER _____

AUDITOR/WITNESS _____

INVESTIGATOR/PHYSICIAN REPRESENTATIVE _____

FIGURE 10.1 Outline for a consent form for documenting a person's informed consent to serve as a subject in a research project. (From Purtile, R.D., and Cassel, C.K., Ethical Dimensions in the Health Professions. Philadelphia: W.B. Saunders (1981).

UTILIZATION OF DATA FROM
RESEARCH IN WHICH SUBJECTS WERE ABUSED

Is it ethical to utilize data from research in which subjects were abused, particularly from that in which they were knowingly abused? Perhaps the most extreme, contemporary example of such data would that gathered in Nazi Germany during World War II which motivated the development of the Nuremberg Code (see Appendix B). Each of us must answer this question for ourself. The following comment by Dr. Tomas Radil-Weiss, a psychiatrist and head of the Section on Neurophysiology of the Czechoslovak Academy of Sciences, who was imprisoned at Auschwitz Concentration Camp when he was 14 years old may be helpful when doing so:

> The second world war ended many years ago. Most of those who survived the stay at the German concentration camp at Auschwitz have already died of the consequences of their imprisonment; those still alive are already in the last third of their life. Is there any point to returning to the experiences of those days? Consideration of the mental hygiene of former prisoners cautions us that perhaps we should not do it. *But consideration of the general interest holds that we are not entitled to ignore any knowledge that can contribute to social development — including medicine and psychology — even if acquired under unspeakably awful conditions* [italics mine] (Radil-Weiss, 1983, p. 259).

The utilization of such data may allow a little good to come from the suffering of those research subjects who have been abused physically or psychologically, purposefully or through negligence.

RESEARCH FRAUD AND MISCONDUCT

A researcher should avoid engaging in behavior that would be likely to be labeled by peers as fraud or misconduct. A researcher not only has an ethical-legal obligation to do so, but also a personal one—i.e., to preserve his or her reputation.

What types of research-related behavior are likely to be labeled by peers as fraud or misconduct? The type that probably would be most likely to be so labeled is fabricating or plagiarizing data. Such behavior has been reported to be extremely rare, but perhaps not as rare as was thought 10 years ago (Hilgartner, 1990). Other types that, while less serious, are almost certainly more widespread include the following:

> listing "honorary authors" who contribute nothing substantive to publications that bear their names, failing to mention that a paper relied on

historical controls, neglecting to disclose conflict of interest when reviewing manuscripts, giving the work of coauthors only a cursory review before "signing off" on it, publishing the same data repeatedly without notifying journal editors, or using misleading statistical techniques. There is also concern about researchers nonrandomly assigning patients in supposedly random clinical trials, and even about researchers handling data negligently (Hilgartner, 1990, p. 2).

While there has been considerable debate about whether these practices should be labeled scientific misconduct, there is agreement that they are undesirable and should be avoided (see Hilgartner, 1990). For additional information about them, see Altman & Melcher (1983), Bailar (1986), Croll (1984), and Stewart & Feder (1987).

Chapter XI

SERVING AS AN EXPERT WITNESS

A speech-language pathologist or audiologist can be asked to testify as either an ordinary or an expert witness at a civil or criminal court proceeding or at a hearing. The hearing would be likely to be conducted under the auspices of an administrative agency such as a state department of public instruction or a local school board. An example would be a *due-process hearing* convened by a local school board to comply with certain requirements of Public Law 94-142 (see Appendix C).

An *ordinary ("fact") witness* "testifies to what he [or she] has seen, heard, or otherwise observed" (Black, 1968, p. 1178). An audiologist might be asked to testify about the hearing of a person that he or she had tested. Or a speech-language pathologist might be asked to testify about the therapy that he or she had used with a client. Ordinary witnesses testify about events they have observed—their role usually is to provide rather than evaluate evidence. Their only special qualifications are that they were present when an event occurred and that they are willing and able to describe what they observed.

Expert witnesses, on the other hand, both provide and evaluate evidence. Their special qualifications are that they possess "particular knowledge, wisdom, skill, or information regarding subject matter under consideration, acquired by study, investigation, observation, practice or experience and not likely to be possessed by the ordinary layman or inexperienced person" (Black, 1968, p. 688) and that they have "acquired ability to deduce correct inferences from hypothetical stated facts, or from facts involving scientific or technical knowledge" (Black, 1968, p. 688). They can assist the judge, the jury, and the attorney who retains them in performing their functions, particularly with regard to dealing with subject matter that requires more than a lay-person's knowledge to evaluate and/or comprehend.

Expert witnesses may or may not testify in a court or at a hearing. If they do not do so, they may testify in a deposition prior to the trial or hearing or they may merely function as consultants to the attorneys who retain them. An expert witness's remarks, conclusions, and opinions ordinarily are protected when he or she is functioning as a consultant — they do not have to be communicated to the opposing attorney. Of course, the attorney who retains the expert may do so if he or she feels that communicating it is likely to help his or her client (e.g., encourage the other party to drop the suit or accept an out-of-court settlement).

When expert witnesses give depositions and/or testify in court or at a hearing, their remarks, conclusions, and opinions ordinarily are not protected and will be *painstakingly scrutinized* by the opposing attorney. The opposition will attempt — through the process of *cross-examination* — to reduce the positive impact of their testimony on the judge and jury by casting doubt on their credibility as experts and/or the validity of their conclusions and opinions. The attorney who retains the expert witness will attempt to establish the expert's credibility and the validity of his or her testimony sufficiently strongly so that even after cross-examination the testimony will have the desired impact on the judge and jury.

SUBJECTS ABOUT WHICH SPEECH-LANGUAGE PATHOLOGISTS AND AUDIOLOGISTS HAVE TESTIFIED AS EXPERT WITNESSES

Expert witnesses function in both civil and criminal court proceedings and in hearings. Speech-language pathologists and audiologists have testified as experts in all three types of proceedings. Some of the subjects about which they have been asked to testify are indicated in this section.

Criminal Court Proceedings

In criminal cases speech-language pathologists and audiologists have probably most often been asked to provide expert testimony (1) to establish the *competency* of a defendant to be tried and (2) to confirm the *identification* of a defendant.

Under our legal system, a person ordinarily cannot be tried and convicted for committing a crime unless he or she is judged *legally competent.* An aspect of being legally competent is being able to comprehend what is transpiring during one's trial. "In the United States of America it is a firmly established principle of law that a person cannot be put on trial if his [or her] condition is such that he [or she] will not be able to understand the proceedings and make a proper defense" (Meyers, 1968, p. 130). This ordinarily would be the case for a person who is deaf, and unable to speak, and unable to comprehend sign language or any other language system. It also could be the case for a severe receptive or global aphasic. The role of the expert witness in such an instance would be to assess the communicative competency of the defendant and to testify about it in a deposition and/or in court.

The prosecution has introduced as evidence in some criminal cases an *identification of a defendant* based on the person's speech, voice, or fluency (e.g., whether or not he or she is a stutterer—see Bloodstein, 1988 and Shirkey, 1987). A prosecutor may introduce such evidence, for example, to prove that a defendant made certain obscene telephone calls. In such cases the prosecutor may attempt to introduce as evidence an acoustic analysis of a recorded speech sample known as a *voice print* (Block, 1975). The identification of persons from their speech, voice, or fluency patterns is controversial, and speech-language pathologists have been asked to testify as expert witnesses both supporting (for the prosecution) and questioning (for the defense) the validity and reliability of such identification.

Civil Court Proceedings

In civil cases speech-language pathologists and audiologists have most often been asked to provide expert testimony on (1) competency, (2) personal injury, and (3) custody of minors in divorce cases (Fox, 1978).

Speech-language pathologists and audiologists have been asked to testify about a person's *competency* in civil as well as criminal court proceedings. In a civil case they would testify about a person's competency to manage his or her financial and other affairs rather than competency to stand trial. Some members of an aphasic's family, for example, may seek to have him declared incompetent to manage his financial affairs (Rada, Porch, and Kellner, 1975). A speech-language pathologist could be asked to testify as an expert in such an instance by the attorney representing either the family or the aphasic.

In *personal injury* cases the court must establish the extent of the injury and the prognosis for improvement before it can determine how much compensation (i.e., compensatory damages) the injured party should be awarded. Such cases include proceedings for malpractice (see Chapter 6) and worker's compensation. Speech-language pathologists and audiologists have been asked to examine a plaintiff's speech, language, and/or hearing and to testify as an expert about the extent to which the plaintiff's communicative disorder is handicapping to him or her and the likelihood that the degree of handicap will be lessened in the future. An audiologist, for example, may be asked to testify as an expert about the hearing of a person who is seeking *worker's compensation* for a hearing loss that she claims resulted from exposure to high levels of noise at her place of employment. Or a speech-language pathologist may be asked to testify as an expert about the aphonia of a person who is suing an anesthetist for *malpractice* because he claims that the anesthetist damaged his vocal folds when he passed a tube between them during a surgical procedure.

A speech-language pathologist or audiologist may be asked to testify as an expert in cases concerned with the *custody of minors following divorce.* Family courts are supposed to award custody of minor children to the parent who can best meet their needs. If a child has a communicative disorder that requires treatment, one factor the court probably will consider when deciding on custody is the ability of each parent to make it possible for the child to receive necessary therapy. If one parent, for example, planned to reside in a rural area where therapy would not be readily available and the other planned to reside in an urban one where it would be readily available, the court (at least with regard to this factor) would tend to favor the "urban" rather than the "rural" parent. In custody cases speech-language pathologists and audiologists would ordinarily testify about such matters as the therapy and special educational needs of the child and the likelihood of being able to meet these needs where each parent plans to reside. They might also testify about the ability of each parent to cope with problems arising from the child's communicative disorder. One parent, for example, may be able to understand almost all of a dysarthric child's speech and the other very little of it.

Administrative Agency Hearings

Administrative agencies conduct hearings that are somewhat similar in format to court proceedings. In fact, they are sometimes referred to as *quasi-judicial* proceedings. One feature they share with court proceedings is the use of expert witnesses. A speech-language pathologist or audiologist is probably more likely to be asked to testify as an expert at a hearing than at a civil or criminal court proceeding.

Speech-language pathologists and audiologists have frequently testified as experts at hearings associated with Public Law 94-142, which mandates local school districts to meet the special educational needs of all children residing in the geographical area(s) that they serve. If the parents of a child feel that their school district is not adequately meeting his or her needs, they can request a hearing at which they are likely to be represented by an attorney. If the child has a communicative disorder and the parents question the appropriateness of the intervention the school district is providing, their attorney may ask a speech-language pathologist or audiologist to examine the child and testify as an expert about the child's special educational needs and the services required. Or the attorney representing the school district may make such a request in an attempt to establish that it is adequately meeting the child's needs.

FUNCTIONING AS AN EXPERT WITNESS

This section presents some guidelines for functioning as an expert witness in a court proceeding or hearing. They were synthesized from several sources intended for preparing physicians to serve as expert witnesses. The order in which they are presented in not necessarily related to their importance. They are intended to supplement rather than substitute for a pretrial (or prehearing) conference with the attorney requesting the services.

Projecting an Appropriate Image

The impact that an expert's testimony has on a judge and jury is determined not only by what he or she says, but also by his or her conduct while testifying. If they perceive the expert a someone who is both *knowledgeable* about the subject and *confident* about the accuracy of the testimony, they will tend to give the testimony more weight than they will if they feel that he or she is not knowledgeable about the subject or not confident about the accuracy of some of his or her testimony. Also, if the expert does not *dress appropriately* (i.e., in a manner consistent with expectations about how an "expert" should dress) or *communicate well,* his or her testimony may be given less credibility than it deserves. While it is unfortunate that the manner in which expert witnesses conduct themselves can profoundly influence the impact of their testimony on a judge and jury, it is nevertheless a fact of life with which they must contend. Consequently, those testifying as experts have to conduct themselves in a manner that will maximize the probability that a judge and jury will give appropriate weight to their testimony.

A number of variables can influence the image that an expert witness projects, including the following:

1. The amount of *eye contact* the expert has with the judge and jury (particularly the latter). Having frequent eye contact with them while testifying ordinarily will enhance a witness's image.

2. The extent to which the expert can maintain his or her *composure.* The more successful the expert witness is at reflecting confidence and assurance while testifying, the more credence the judge and jury are likely to give to the testimony. Consequently, during cross-examination the opposing attorney is likely to attempt to get the expert to lose his or her composure.

3. The extent to which the witness establishes his or her *qualifications* to testify as an expert. The more successful he or she is at establishing these qualifications, the more credible the judge and jury will tend to regard the testimony. The opposing attorney may attempt to nullify the testimony by questioning to the witness's qualifications to testify as an expert about the matter at hand.

4. The extent to which the witness succeeds at *communicating* with the judge and jury. Some experts attempt to impress a jury by using many esoteric scientific terms. This is a questionable strategy. A jury is more likely to be persuaded by an expert who attempts to communicate with them in language they can understand. An expert witness should assume that the members of the jury know nothing about his or her field of expertise and take on a responsibility to communicate findings and opinions to them in language they can understand. Obviously, while doing this he or she should be careful not to appear to be talking down to them.

5. The extent to which the expert has *reviewed the testimony* with the attorney who retained him or her. If the attorney either is unaware of or does not understand what the expert can say that may be helpful to the client, the attorney may not ask the appropriate questions during *direct examination.* An expert witness ordinarily testifies during direct examination by answering a series of questions asked by the attorney who retained him or her. If all of the questions that need to be answered in order to present the testimony are not asked, then the expert's testimony may not have the positive impact on the judge and jury that it deserves. The attorney may ask the expert to formulate a series of questions, the answers to which would allow the testimony to be presented in a relatively complete, clear, and organized manner.

A *second reason* why the expert should review the testimony with the attorney is to indicate to him or her how the opposing attorney is likely to attempt to refute it during cross-examination. If the attorney is aware of this, he or she will probably be better prepared to lessen the negative impact of cross-examination on it by asking the expert appropriate questions during *redirect examination.*

A *third reason* why the expert should meet with the attorney prior to appearing in court is to make certain that the attorney knows enough about the expert's background to convince the judge and jury that he or she is qualified to testify as an expert about the matter at hand. The attorney, to establish the credibility of the expert, asks a series of questions at the beginning of the *direct examination.* (There is a representative set of such questions elsewhere in the chapter.) The expert witness can be helpful to the attorney by reviewing these questions to make certain they will allow him or her to present the information necessary to establish credibility as an expert.

6. The *directness* with which the expert witness answers questions. If the expert is perceived by the judge and jury as being evasive or defensive when answering questions, the potential positive impact of the testimony on them is likely to be reduced. An expert witness must be particularly careful not to appear evasive when asked by the opposing attorney (during cross-examination) to answer yes or no to a question that the expert believes cannot be adequately answered with a simple yes or no. In such a situation an expert witness is permitted to appeal to the judge. The judge may allow the witness to give a fuller answer, but if not, the expert *should not argue about it.* The attorney who retained the expert can provide him or her an opportunity to answer more fully during the redirect examination.

7. The *respect* the expert shows for the judge and jury. The judge is the "boss" of the court and the expert witness should always show respect. Failure to do so can adversely affect the image that the members of the jury have of the expert since they tend to expect witnesses to be respectful of the judge. It can also result in the expert being held in *contempt of court.*

8. Whether the jury believes the expert is *being paid for testifying.* An expert witness ordinarily receives a fee—not for the testimony, but for his or her time, professional knowledge, and services for studying the facts of the case and formulating opinions based on them. If the opposing attorney (during cross-examination) can make the jury believe that

the expert testified as he or she did because of the fee received, they are apt to give little weight to the testimony.

Testifying

An expert witness's testimony ordinarily can be divided into four parts. The first part consists of answers to questions about personal background and experience, which are asked by the attorney who retained him or her. Its purpose is to establish credibility to testify as an expert about the matter at hand.

The second part consists of answers to questions about the case, which are asked by the attorney who retained him or her. These questions and answers are the "meat" of the expert's *direct testimony*.

The third part consists of answers to questions about the direct testimony, which are asked by the opposing attorney. These questions are likely to deal both with the expert's qualifications to testify as an expert about the matter at hand and with the expert's testimony about the case. This part is referred to as *cross-examination*. It is an attempt to nullify the expert's direct testimony by suggesting to the jury that he or she is not qualified to testify as an expert about the matter at hand, or that his or her interpretations (opinions) are not the only possible ones, or both of these.

The fourth part consists of answers to questions about the expert's testimony during cross-examination, that are asked by the attorney who retained him or her. The attorney's objective during this part (which is referred to as the *redirect examination*) is to reestablish the qualifications of the witness and to establish that the interpretations (opinions) given in testimony are more viable than those suggested by the opposing attorney during cross-examination.

Some guidelines for testifying as an expert during each of these four parts are presented in the following paragraphs.

Being Qualified as an Expert. The first task of the attorney who retained the expert witness is to establish during direct examination that the witness is competent to testify as an expert about the matter at hand. If the attorney is successful, the trial judge will rule that the witness is competent to do so. The attorney will then go on to the substantive part of the direct examination.

To qualify the witness as an expert, the attorney asks a series of questions. The following series, which was abstracted from several sources

(Imwinkelried, 1980; Jeans, 1975; Mauet, 1980; & Moenssens, 1973), is representative:

Q: Will you state your name, please?
Q: Will you state your business address, please?
Q: What is your business occupation?
Q: What is your present title?
Q: For how long have you been employed in this occupation?
Q: Will you briefly describe, please, the subject matter of this occupation?
Q: Do you specialize within this occupation?
Q: What is your specialty?
Q: What is it concerned with?
Q: How long have you been in practice in this specialty?
Q: What is your formal education?
Q: What undergraduate school did you attend?
Q: What degree did you obtain there?
Q: What was your major field of study?
Q: What graduate school(s) did you attend?
Q: What degree(s) did you obtain there?
Q: What was your major field of study?
Q: What postgraduate training have you received?
Q: Are you licensed (or certified) to practice this occupation?
Q: By whom was this license (or certification) awarded?
Q: For how long have you had it?
Q: What positions have you held since the completion of your formal training?
Q: For how long did you hold each?
Q: To what professional organizations do you belong?
Q: What are the qualifications for becoming a member of these organizations?
Q: What offices and committee assignments have you held in these organizations?
Q: Have you taught courses in your specialty?
Q: Where?
Q: Have you published articles or books?
Q: How many articles have you published?
Q: In what scientific journals did they appear?
Q: How many books have you published?

Q: What are the titles of your books?
Q: What topics did you discuss in your articles and books?
Q: Have you ever testified in court as an expert witness?
Q: What subjects have you testified on?
Q: How many clients diagnosed as having . . . have you treated?
Q: Have you ever previously evaluated a client for (e.g., competency to manage his financial affairs)?
Q: How many times have you performed such an evaluation?

The specific questions that an expert witness will be asked depend on his or her background and experience and the subject matter about which he or she will be testifying. If, for example, the expert has not published any articles or books, question pertaining to publication will not be asked.

The opposing attorney is entitled to cross-examine the witness about these qualifications. He or she may do so at this stage of the proceeding or wait until the direct examination has been completed.

An expert witness should not feel compelled to answer questions immediately after they are asked; it is wise to avoid appearing either too willing or reluctant. When answering, he or she should be brief and to the point, not volunteering extra information but answering only the questions asked. If a question is not clearly phrased, the witness should not hesitate to ask the attorney to clarify it. If the attorney makes an inaccurate remark or interprets testimony in a way that is not completely accurate, the expert should make a correction; otherwise, the opposing attorney probably will.

Direct Examination. After the trial judge rules that the witness is competent to testify as an expert, the attorney begins the questioning about the matter that is to be the subject of testimony. Some questions are likely to be *fact* questions about the person who has the communicative disorder and the services the person has received. Others will be *opinion* questions. The witness may be asked to give an opinion based on the facts (evidence) in the case or a series of assumptions. The latter involves answering a *hypothetical question.* An answer to such a question should conform to the facts that are substantiated in the evidence of the case.

An expert witness should *avoid bringing written records* to court if at all possible. When records are used while testifying, they become part of the evidence. The opposing attorney can examine them, comment on them, and read from them to the judge and jury. An expert witness would be unwise, therefore, to bring any written records that he or she would not want read aloud in court.

Ordinarily an expert witness is permitted to use *exhibits and demonstrations* to clarify points that might otherwise be confusing to a jury. Exhibits can vary from anatomical diagrams (e.g., of the ear) to audiotapes or videotapes (e.g., to demonstrate the magnitude of the person's communicative disorder). Juries tend to be fascinated by demonstrations and exhibits that show the functions of the human body. The expert witness may request a blackboard if writing or drawing on it will help make certain points. While presenting exhibits and demonstrations the expert witness should face the jury and address it directly.

Cross-Examination. The opposing attorney is given the opportunity to cross-examine the expert witness after the direct examination has been completed. He or she will attempt to *reduce or nullify* any positive impact that the expert's testimony has had on the jury. There are several strategies that may be used for this purpose. One is to attempt raise questions in the minds of the jury members about the witness's qualifications to testify as an expert *about the matter at hand.* If, for example, a speech-language pathologist had testified as an expert about aphasia, the opposing attorney may attempt to prove that the clinician's previous experience with cases of aphasia had been quite limited and, hence, the correctness of his or her opinions is uncertain. Merely raising questions in the minds of the jury members about the correctness of certain aspects of the expert's testimony can significantly reduce or nullify its positive impact on them.

Another strategy that the opposing attorney may use to reduce or nullify to positive impact of an expert's testimony is to raise questions in the minds of the jury members about whether the expert was *paid to testify in the manner that he or she did.* The attorney would ask the witness if he or she was paid a fee for testifying? If the witness answered "yes," the attorney would attempt to use this to case doubt on the impartiality of the testimony. (This point is discussed in greater depth elsewhere in this chapter.) The attorney may also attempt to cast doubt on the witness's impartiality by asking how many times he or she has testified as an expert. If the answer indicates a relatively large number of times, the attorney is likely to attempt to convince the jury that the expert is a "gun for hire."

A third strategy an opposing attorney may use of reduce or nullify the positive impact of an expert's testimony is to convince the members of the jury that the expert's opinions *are not the only possible viable ones.* The attorney could attempt to do this in several ways. He or she might attempt to get the expert witness to admit that (1) the interpretations and opinions put forth are not the only ones that would be consistent with the evidence and/or (2) the expert cannot be completely certain about the accuracy of his or her testimony. Also, attorneys often introduce into evidence the testimony of their own expert witnesses which contradicts that of the ones for the other side. By so doing, they convey the message to the members of the jury that *experts disagree.* Such a message, obviously, would tend to reduce the positive impact of an expert's testimony.

The expert witness and the opposing attorney are *adversaries* during cross-examination. The attorney has a single objective—to induce the expert to behave (verbally and/or nonverbally) in a manner that will reduce or eliminate any positive impact that his or her testimony has had on the members of the jury. And the expert witness also should have a single objective—to project to the members of the jury an "image" that will not reduce any positive impact that his or her testimony has had on them and will possibly *enhance it.*

During cross-examination an attorney may attempt to influence a witness's behavior in various ways that could reduce the positive impact of his or her testimony on the jury, including the following:

1. To cause the witness to become angry and counterattack. If the attorney is successful, the members of the jury are likely to perceive the witness as being *less dignified* than they originally thought, which could reduce the weight that they give to his or her testimony.

2. To cause the witness to lower his or her guard by behaving in a friendly fashion. The opposing attorney behaves in a manner that the witness interprets as *relaxed and friendly.* This is designed to cause the witness to lower any defenses and say things that will weaken the testimony. When the opposing attorney comes on in this fashion, the expert witness should *raise* rather than lower his or her guard.

3. To intimidate the witness. A cross-examiner might grimly shuffle a batch of papers while approaching the witness stand to frighten the witness into thinking that they contain evidence damaging to his or her testimony. Of the cross-examiner might write down some of the witness's responses in a very conspicuous manner, thereby suggesting that ammunition to destroy the testimony is being collected. If the attorney is successful and the witness exhibits overt signs of fright, not only might the expert's credibility with the members of the jury be reduced, but the

expert could say things (because of not thinking clearly) that would weaken the testimony.

4. To cause the witness to agree that an opinion may be a *speculation*. If an expert witness agrees with a cross-examiner that a particular opinion may be a speculation, the members of the jury may interpret this response to mean the opinion is mere guess work. If a cross-examiner suggests that an opinion is speculation, the witness should indicate that it is not speculation, but is based on "reasonable professional certainty and in accordance with scientific probability" (Sanbar, 1977).

5. To cause the witness to *disparage the expert testimony for the opposite side*. To do so could cause some members of the jury to lose respect for the witness, which could result in their giving his or her testimony less weight than they would have otherwise. If an expert witness during cross-examination is asked to explain the conflicting expert testimony for the opposite side, he or she can answer by saying, "I am sure _____ is a competent professional, but I simply do not agree on this particular issue" (Sanbar, 1977).

6. To cause the witness to answer a question with a "yes" that should be answered with a "no." A cross-examiner may ask an expert witness a series of questions at a relatively rapid rate, all of which call for the answer "yes" and then ask one that should be answered "no." Because of the rhythm the witness has developed to say "yes," he or she may end up saying "yes" when meaning to say "no."

An expert's testimony in some instances will end following cross-examination. If this is the case, the judge will indicate it. He or she should not leave the witness stand before being told to do so by the judge. It is important to maintain dignity when leaving the witness stand—never making any obvious victory signs or signs of relief, and do not grin broadly as a sign of triumph, nor run away from the stand with unseemly haste (Sanbar, 1977).

Redirect Examination. The attorney who retained the expert will in some instances want to ask additional questions to "repair the damage" that was done during cross-examination. The points that should be kept in mind when answering such questions are those that were mentioned in the section on direct examination.

For further information about testifying as an expert witness see Kramer and Ambruster (1982), Machovec (1987), and Shapiro (1984).

THE EXPERT WITNESS FEE

An expert witness is ordinarily paid a fee to compensate for time and testimony-related expenses. He or she should seek to be paid an hourly rate rather than a lump sum fee. The hours that are compensated should include not only those spent in court (or at hearings) but also those incurred in making out reports, attending pretrial (or prehearing) conferences, and gathering data (including examining the person who has the communicative disorder). The expenses should include transportation costs, hotel rooms, meals, tips, time spent on the telephone, and consultations (Sanbar, 1977). He or she should carefully record and, if possible, document both the amount of time spent on a case and the expenses incurred.

It is unethical for an expert witness to enter into an agreement that makes the fee contingent on the outcome of the trial. However, it would not be unethical for him or her to agree to serve without guarantee of payment (Sanbar, 1977).

To avoid misunderstandings an expert witness should have a written agreement (contract) with the attorney who retains him or her. It should specify the amount to be paid, by whom, and when. This agreement should include a provision assuring compensation for preparations and services provided in the event that a settlement is reached before the suit is heard by a court.

Chapter XII

LOBBYING FOR LEGISLATIVE CHANGE

The 1991 Code of Ethics of the American Speech-Language-Hearing Association (see Appendix D) requires speech-language pathologists and audiologists to "hold paramount the welfare of persons served professionally." In addition, it charges them to "expand services to persons with speech, language, and hearing problems." These injunctions imply that speech-language pathologists and audiologists have a responsibility to the communicatively handicapped that extends beyond their own caseloads, a responsibility that includes doing everything possible to insure that persons requiring speech, language, or hearing services will be able to receive them. One of the main reasons why communicatively handicapped persons may not receive needed services is *lack of funding*. The clinical services received by the majority of communicatively handicapped persons at this time are not paid for directly by them or their families. They are paid for by a *third party*, in most instances a governmental administrative agency. These agencies (including local school boards, state departments of public instruction, and the federal Social Security Administration) are able to provide the funding because they have been allocated funds for the purpose by municipal, state, or federal legislatures. Such legislatures have the ability to maintain a given level of funding for speech, language, and hearing services, to increase this level of funding, or to reduce it. The level of funding they allocate for such services is partially determined by the arguments that are presented to them for increasing, reducing, or maintaining the existing level. These arguments are presented to them by persons functioning as *lobbyists*.

After 1972, the frequency with which speech-language pathologists and audiologists functioned as lobbyists for the communicatively handicapped increased considerably. This increase in activity on the federal level was mainly due to the creation of the American Speech-Language-Hearing Association's *Congressional Action Contact (CAC) Network* in that year (Congressional Action Contact Network Handbook, 1991). A member of the Association is assigned to each member of Congress (each senator and each representative) to lobby the legislator on bills that are or will be under consideration. The member assigned is a *constituent* of the legislator. Some state associations now maintain similar networks for lobbying members of their legislature (Wolf, Powell, & Montgomery, 1989) and two-thirds of them have lobbyists or legislative agents who represent the members' interests in the state capitol (Browne, 1991). "All state associations need member support to assist in [legislative and regulatory] grass-roots activities" (Browne, 1991, p. 40).

My objectives in this chapter are to increase your awareness of the need for lobbying "to promote the welfare of" the communicatively handicapped and to provide you with some practical information about how to do it. The information is presented in the hope that it will motivate you to do it, possibly by participating in ASHA's Congressional Action Contact Network or a comparable network maintained by your state association. I have been involved with ASHA's CAC Network since its inception and feel that the time I've invested has been well spent.

WHAT IS A LOBBYIST?

Any person who *consciously* attempts to influence the activities (particularly votes) of legislators can be regarded as a lobbyist. The legislator that he or she attempts to influence may be a member of Congress or of a state or municipal legislature. Lobbyists ordinarily attempt to influence legislators by making them aware of their position on particular bills and of the need for certain legislation. An example of the latter would be the lobbying done by many members of state associations to have licensure bills for professionals in our field introduced in their legislatures. A lobbyist may be paid (by an organization) or a volunteer. He or she may use any of a number of approaches to influence legislators, including (1) writing letters or sending telegrams (or mailgrams), (2) engaging in face-to-face discussions to explain in detail the reasons for positions being advocated, (3) testifying before legislative committees, and/or (4) preparing briefs, memorandums, legislative analyses, and draft legislation for use by legislative committees and individual legislators. Each of these is discussed elsewhere in this chapter.

Lobbyists are granted the right to attempt to influence legislators in the *First Amendment* to the U.S. Constitution:

Congress shall make no laws ... abridging the freedom of speech, or of the press, or the right of the people peaceably to assemble, *and to petition the Government for a redress of grievances* [italics mine].

This right is based largely on the guarantees of free speech and the peoples' right "to petition the Government for a redress of grievances." Lobbyists have influenced legislation on federal, state, and municipal levels since the founding of our country (Schriftgiesser, 1951; *The Washington Lobby,* 1971).

Ethical lobbyists (as opposed to unscrupulous ones) perform an *important function* in the legislative process. They speak knowledgeably for various economic, commercial, minority, and other interests. Legislators are unlikely to be highly knowledgeable about the subject matter of all the bills on which they are expected to vote. To cast an informed vote on a bill, they must understand the various implications of its being passed and becoming a law. Lobbyists representing *special interest groups* that have different points of view about a particular bill can help legislators understand its ramifications by presenting them with arguments and evidence supporting their groups point of view. (Individuals having strong points of view about particular bills can do the same thing—in fact, when doing so they are functioning as lobbyists.) Hence, lobbyists can provide legislators with information that will allow them to cast more informed votes than they probably would be able to cast otherwise. In a sense lobbyists advocating various positions on an issue perform a similar service for *legislators* that attorneys representing plaintiff and defendant do in a trial for a *judge and jury*—that is, presenting the strongest case they can for their side, thereby maximizing the probability that an appropriate decision will be reached.

Most organizations (associations) have as an aspect of their mandate the encouragement of legislation consistent with the special interests shared by their members. People join an organization presumably because it allows them to interact with others who share one of their special interests: The organization, thereby, becomes a credible "spokesperson" for persons having that special interest. It may retain a professional lobbyist (or lobbyists) to monitor pending legislation and, where appropriate, present its points of view on such legislation. Or it may rely on some of its members who are not professional lobbyists to perform these functions. Or it may rely on a combination of professional lobbyists and member volunteers. The American Speech-Language-Hearing Association uses a combination approach (*Congressional Action Contact Network Handbook*, 1991). The organization employs professional lobbyists to monitor pending legislation and present its point of view to legislators and members of their staffs. It also uses member volunteers (CAC Network) to present its points of view on pending legislation to members of Congress when the staff of its Governmental Affairs Department believes that doing so could be helpful.

An organization (such as ASHA) through its lobbying activities can *indirectly* promote the welfare of its members by promoting the welfare of those who are consumers of the goods and services that its members provide. If the American Speech-Language-Hearing Association, for example, supports legislation that would provide increased services for a segment of the communicatively handicapped population, it also is encouraging an increased demand for the services provided by its members and, hence, additional employment opportunities for them. The motivation of the organization to lobby for the welfare of those who consume the goods and/or services provided by its members, therefore, is partially altruistic and partially self-serving.

APPROACHES USED BY LOBBYISTS TO INFLUENCE LEGISLATORS

Lobbyists, both professional and volunteer, as I indicated previously, have used a number of approaches (singly or in combination) to influence legislators' votes. These include (1) "bribery," (2) writing letters or sending telegrams (or mailgrams), (3) engaging in face-to-face discussions to explain in detail the reasons for positions being advocated, (4) testifying before legislative committees, and/or (5) preparing briefs, memorandums, legislative analyses, and draft legislation for use by legislative committees and individual legislators. Some implications of each of these approaches are indicated in this section.

"Bribery"

Bribery is one of the oldest approaches that lobbyists have used to influence legislators. In its most blatant form, it involves the payment of money (or its equivalent) to legislators in exchange for their supporting or not supporting a particular bill. The ABSCAM scandal of the early 1980s in which an FBI agent posing as a lobbyist offered bribes to a number of members of Congress (which they accepted) for their support on a particular bill indicates that attempted bribery in its most blatant form can still occur. This approach does have a serious limitation other than being expensive—i.e., it is a *crime* for a lobbyist to offer a bribe and for a legislator to accept it. A reputable organization, such as ASHA, would of course be highly unlikely to try such an approach.

The form of bribery in which a legislator is paid directly for a vote probably occurs relatively infrequently because it is a crime. There is, however, an indirect form of bribery practiced by special interest groups, that is not a crime and that appears to be quite wide-spread: i.e., making contributions through their political action committees (PACs) to the *campaign funds* of certain persons running for election or reelection to a legislature (municipal, state, or federal). If they are elected, they may feel obligated to the special interest groups who supported them financially, which could influence their votes on certain legislation. ASHA, through its Political Action Committee (ASHA–PAC), contributes to the campaign funds of some persons who are running for election or reelection to Congress (ASHA–PAC: A visible influence, 1988; ASHA–PAC wants effective leaders, 1990); Koenigknecht, 1990b).

There is another form of "bribery" used by lobbyists that ordinarily is not regarded as being such. An example would be a lobbyist arranging to have a legislator address the special interest group that he or she represents. The legislator probably would receive some media coverage for his or her presentation and an honorarium. A state association that is seeking passage of a licensure bill may invite a state legislator whom they feel might be willing to sponsor the bill to be the luncheon speaker at their annual convention.

Writing Letters and Sending Telegrams

A letter or telegram from a constituents to a legislator which communicates his or her point of view on a bill based on professional expertise and experience can influence how the legislator will vote on it. The likelihood that it will do so is, in part, a function of how it is written. It should be "personal—clearly handwritten or typed. Nothing looks worse to a legislator than an obvious, orchestrated campaign. There is no substitute for a carefully worded, thoughtful letter [or telegram] from a constituent" (*Congressional Action Contact Network Handbook,* 1991).

The following are some DOs and DON'Ts that ASHA recommends should be followed when corresponding with a legislator (*Congressional Action Contact Network Handbook,* 1991):

The Fundamental DOs

DO address . . . [the legislator] properly.

Proper form for addressing . . . members of Congress

Honorable (full name)
U.S. House of Representatives
Washington, DC 20515

Dear Representative:

Honorable (full name)
U.S. Senate
Washington, DC 20510

Dear Senator:

DO write legibly. (Typed letters are preferable, but handwritten letters are acceptable if they are readable.)

DO use your own words and personal or business stationery.

DO be brief and to the point. Discuss only single issues or related issues in each letter.

DO identify your subject clearly; give the name of the legislation or the bill number if you know it.

DO state your reason for writing. Cite personal experiences and show how the issue would effect you, the professions, the population you serve, and the district the legislator represents.

DO draw attention to the personal connection you may have with the legislator or a time you met.

DO ask the legislator to state his/her position on the issue when replying to your letter. As a constituent you are entitled to know.

DO request specific action; tell the legislator what you want him or her to do.

DO be sure to include your address and sign your name legibly. If you have family, business, or political connections related to the issue, explain them. They may serve as identification when your point of view is considered.

DO feel free to write if you have a question or problem dealing with procedures of governmental departments. Congressional offices often can help you cut through red tape or give advice that can save you time and effort.

DO include pertinent editorials from local papers.

DO time your letters for maximum effect. Write early in a session when bills are introduced if you have ideas about an issue that you would like to see incorporated into legislation. If . . . [a legislator] is a member of a committee to which it has been referred, write when the committee begins hearings. If the legislator is not a member of the committee handling the bill, write just before the bill comes to the floor for debate and vote.

DO write the chairman or chairwoman, or members of the committee holding hearings on legislation that interests you, especially if you have facts that could influence his or her thinking.

DO write to say you approve, not just to complain or oppose. Public officials hear mostly from constituents who oppose their actions.

DO thank ... [them] if they have taken a position or cast a vote that you think is right on a particular issue. Knowing that constituents approve of their actions is important to legislators and will help reaffirm the position when the issue comes up again.

The Fundamental DON'Ts

DON'T apologize for taking his or her time. If you are brief and to the point, he or she is glad to hear from you.

DON'T be argumentative; you are trying to convince the legislator to incorporate your views into his/her legislative positions.

DON'T be vague. Some letters received in congressional offices are couched in such general terms that they leave Senators/Representatives and their staffs wondering what the writer had in mind.

DON'T try to cover too many issues in a single letter ... It is best to limit the content of your letter to one issue that is particularly pertinent to you. If there are several unrelated issues (e.g., preschool education and biomedical research), it is best to cover them in separate letters. Chances are these issues will be handled by different staff in the congressional office.

DON'T write to your legislator's local district office unless your correspondence deals with a local issue. You will receive a quicker response when you use the Washington, D.C. address. . . .

Face-to-Face Discussions with Legislators

Meeting a legislator personally can be an effective method for communicating your point of view on a bill. The likelihood that your get-together will influence the legislator in the way you desire is, in part, a function of how you conduct yourself prior to and during the session. The following *DOs* and *DON'Ts* for a successful meeting have been suggested by ASHA (*Congressional Action Contact Network Handbook*, 1991):

DOs

DO make an appointment in advance; you will be scheduled for a specific amount of time, and you will be asked what the subject matter is. Be sure to stick to the scheduled amount of time allotted you.

DO be on time for your scheduled appointment. Be prepared to wait.

DO be flexible. If the member cannot meet with you at the scheduled time, reschedule an appointment or meet with the Administrative or Legislative Assistant.

DO be prepared. Present pertinent facts, figures, opinions. Be brief, articulate, and persuasive; get to the point; have material to back up your position.

DO give the legislator a chance to talk; you may be surprised at his/her knowledge and/or questions.

DO keep on the subject of discussion; do not let the conversation stray to other subjects.

DO leave materials that repeat your major points with the staff.

DO get to know the legislator's staff, especially the administrative and/or legislative assistant. Because of the volume and complexity of legislation, Members of Congress rely on their staffs to do research, watch the progress of legislation of interest to constituents, and prepare summaries and recommendations on the various measures. The better informed the aid is, the more complete his recommendations can be for the legislator.

DO follow up your meeting with a letter of thanks; include a summary of the points you made at the meeting.

DO use the proper salutation when meeting with . . . [the legislator] (Senator _____ or Congressman/Congresswoman or Representative _____.)

DON'Ts

DON'T make the meeting too long; offer to sent any additional information that may have been requested by mail.

DON'T give up on the Member because he/she doesn't vote your way on every issue. You don't know what his/her commitments are on many issues. Give him/her the benefit of the doubt.

DON'T argue if the Member doesn't give you a definite positive position. Keep the lines of communication open; if the Member is not on your side today, he/she may be two months from now.

DON'T overlook the staff aids in the office. They can be very influential with the legislator.

Meetings with members of Congress can be set up at their local district offices when the body is in recess. While it is in session they can be scheduled at their office in Washington, D.C.

Testifying Before Legislative Committees

Before a bill is considered by a particular legislative body (such as the Senate or House of Representatives), it ordinarily is considered by a *committee* made up of members of that body. The mandate given to this committee is to conduct a *hearing* to explore the ramifications of the bill thoroughly. Following the hearing, the committee is expected to recommend what action the legislative body should take on the bill. Lobbyists and others representing special interest groups ordinarily are permitted to testify at these hearings. Their testimony consists of arguments, supported by evidence, indicating why they believe (or the group they represent believes) that the bill under consideration should or should not be enacted into law. Those who testify usually are questioned by members of the committee following their formal presentation. (To learn more about the nature of such testimony, watch a House or Senate hearing for several hours on one of the C–SPAN cable television channels.) Officers of the American Speech-Language-Hearing Association and members of its Governmental Affairs Department staff have testified at such hearings. Officers of state associations and lobbyists retained by them have testified at similar hearings conducted by state legislative committees.

Preparing Briefs, Memorandums, Legislative Analyses, and Draft Legislation

Lobbyists often draft documents for the use of individual legislators and legislative committees. Such documents may summarize statistical or other data that support the point of view the lobbyist is advocating. Or they may summarize the organization's position on certain pending legislation. Or they may be *preliminary drafts of bills* that the special interest group wishes to have considered (and hopefully enacted) by a particular legislative body. A state association that wanted a licensure bill for speech-language pathologists and audiologists passed by its state legislature might prepare a preliminary draft of such a bill and then have the person functioning as its lobbyist attempt to locate one or more legislators who would be willing to *sponsor* it. Of course, locating a sponsor (or sponsors) does not guarantee its passage.

FUNCTIONING AS A LOBBYIST

Many speech-language pathologists and audiologists are somewhat intimidated by the thought of contacting one of their state or federal legislators and attempting to influence his or her vote on a bill. Many of us tend to view our state and federal legislators as authority figures who deal only with important issues, and we assume that they are likely to have little interest in the problems of the communicatively handicapped. Unfortunately, if we approach a legislator with this attitude, it could reduce the amount of weight he or she gives our point of view. It is crucial, therefore, that when we function as lobbyists we truly believe that what we have to say is important to the legislator.

Lobbyists can be viewed as *behavior modifiers.* They are seeking to *shape* the behavior of a legislator. Their overall behavioral objective is to have the legislator sponsor a particular bill or vote in a particular way on it. To achieve this objective lobbyists consciously or unconsciously use *principles of behavior modification.* By presenting arguments supported by data they make legislators sympathetic to their points of view and then *positively reinforce* any comments they make which suggest their attitudes are changing in the direction desired.

What are a lobbyists specific behavioral objectives? One is to convince the legislator that because the position being advocated is valid, the legislator should vote in a particular way or sponsor a particular bill. A second objective is to convince the legislator that it would be advantageous to him or her to do so. Even when legislators are convinced that a particular position is valid, they may not support if they feel that doing so could hurt them—for example, by hurting their chances for reelection.

Information about pending legislation affecting the communicatively handicapped can be found in the *Governmental Affairs Review,* which is published by the American Speech-Language-Hearing Association. This publication reviews both federal and state legislative activity. ASHA also published the *Congressional Action Contact Bulletin* which includes information about bills directly or indirectly affecting the communicatively handicapped being considered by the Congress and *The Governmental Affairs Department (GAD) Report* which includes reports about congressional activity and legislation. Information on this topic also is published in the journal *Asha.*

For further practical information about lobbying, see the *Congressional Action Contact Network Handbook* (1991), Browne (1991), Caplan (1983), and Wolpe (1990).

PLAYING AN ADVOCACY ROLE

The focus thus far in this chapter has been on supporting the passage of bills that benefit persons who are communicatively handicapped. After such a bill has been passed, speech-language pathologists and audiologists have the opportunity to assume a new role in relation to it—that of an *advocate.* In this role they would do everything possible to insure that their clients receive the services they are entitled to under the law (for a discussion of some such services see Dubow, 1982). Clients may not receive services to which they are legally entitled unless their clinicians play an advocacy role.

Why might communicatively handicapped persons not receive services to which they are legally entitled? Often they do not know about the existence of governmental programs from which they could obtain needed funding. Furthermore, sometimes they are refused services to which they are entitled by law. A state department of public instruction, for example, could refuse to fund clinical services for children who have only a single articulation error (e.g., a substitution of w/r) even though federal law (P.L. 94-142) can be interpreted to mean that they are entitled to receive such services.

The ethical responsibility mentioned earlier in this chapter to "hold paramount the welfare of persons served professionally" applies to advocacy as well as to lobbying. Holding paramount the welfare of clients implies having a responsibility to do whatever one can to make it possible for them to receive the clinical services they require. Hence, it implies a responsibility to play an advocacy role.

What could a speech-language pathologist or audiologist, as an advocate, do for a client? The answer to this question depends on why the client is not receiving services to which he or she is legally entitled. If the client is unaware of governmental and other programs that could fund these services, the clinician could play an advocacy role by providing him or her with information about them (see Tucker & Goldstein, 1991). To do this he or she must be aware of municipal, state, and federal programs, as well as those of nongovernmental (e.g., service) organizations, that might fund services the client required but could not totally afford.

A speech-language pathologist or audiologist can also play an advocacy role by convincing the administrators of governmental programs that they should fund services they are not currently funding. This assumes that they are interpreting their regulations to mean that certain services needed by communicatively handicapped persons are not covered and, hence, not fundable. The administrators of some medical insurance programs during the 1970s did not provide funding for electronic augmentative communication devices because they did not interpret their regulations concerning the funding of prostheses to include them. Some speech-language pathologists played an advocacy role by convincing them that electronic augmentative communication devices are *prostheses* (i.e., communication prostheses) and consequently were fundable under existing regulations.

Another way that a speech-language pathologist or audiologist can play an advocacy role is by providing information to clients and their families that might assist them in obtaining services (or funding) they have been refused, despite there being entitled to them by law. The assumption is being made here that those who refused to provide the funding or services are aware the client is entitled to them, but they are refusing perhaps because their budget is not adequate to cover all of the services they are supposed to fund. A clinician may be able to *discreetly* give the client or family information that could result in the agency (e.g., a school system) providing the needed services. The word *discretely* is emphasized because an indiscreet clinician could place himself or herself in a position where the employer (e.g., the school system) would be aware that he or she was functioning as an advocate for the client rather than the employer. Obviously, this would not enhance a clinician's job security.

What advice might a clinician give that could assist a client in obtaining services to which he or she is legally entitled, but has been refused? Perhaps the most effective strategy would be for the client to *threaten legal action* (i.e., a civil suit) if the services or funds are not provided. Most government agencies will go to great lengths to avoid such litigation, particularly if they know they will probably lose. It can be very costly to an agency to lose such litigation because if a court decides that they have to provide services they are not currently providing, it would establish a *precedent* that would be likely to result in requests from others for the services. Hence, the agency may view it as potentially less costly to quietly provide the services rather than risk litigation.

Appendix A
REPRESENTATIVE RELEASE FORMS

PERMISSION FOR RELEASE OF INFORMATION

I hereby give my permission for (insert name of institution) to provide information on

_____ to the following:

_____   _____

_____   _____

_____   _____

_____   _____

This information will consist of the following:

_____

_____

_____

_____

Date _____

Signature _____

Check one: _____ Self

                _____ Parent

                _____ Guardian

Form A-1

PERMISSION FOR REQUEST OF INFORMATION

I hereby give permission to the following:

_____

_____

_____

_____

to release information on _____

to (insert name of institution).

Date _____

Signature _____

Check one: _____ Self

_____ Parent

_____ Guardian

Form A-2

```
         PERMISSION FOR VIDEOTAPING AND RECORDING CLINICAL WORK


                               RE: _____


TO:  (insert name of institution)

     Whereas (insert name of institution), in its speech and hearing

habilitation center, wishes to videotape and record therapy sessions and

the clinical work conducted at the center for use by (insert name of

institution), its students, agents, and employees, therefore, the under-

signed hereby grant permission to (insert name of institution) to record

on film, tape, or otherwise the first name, likeness, and performance of

_____ at the habilitation center for the use of

(insert name of institution).  This permission will remain in force and

effect until revoked in writing by the undersigned.

                               Date _____

                               Signature _____

Check one:  _____ Self

            _____ Parent

            _____ Guardian
```

Form A-3

PERMISSION FOR PUBLICATION OF PHOTOGRAPHS

IN PROMOTIONAL LITERATURE (I.E., MODEL RELEASE)

I hereby give (insert name of institution) the absolute right and permission to copyright and/or publish the photographic portraits or pictures of _____ that were taken on _____, 198_. I agree that the photographs become the exclusive property of (insert name of institution) and I waive all rights thereto.

I waive all rights to inspect and/or approve copy that may be used in conjunction with the photographs and the use to which it may be applied.

The photographs -- whole, in part, or composite -- may be used as (insert name of institution) sees fit in the publication of educational and promotional materials and for any other lawful purpose.

Date _____

Signature _____

Check one: _____ Self

_____ Parent

_____ Guardian

Form A-4

PERMISSION FOR PARTICIPATING IN NONTHERAPEUTIC RESEARCH

TITLE OF PROJECT:

I, _____, hereby consent to participate in the
experimental project being conducted by (insert name of institution)
where (insert description of task). I have been told that (insert statement of what subject has been told about potential risks). I understand
that I may choose to discontinue participation in the project at any
time if I so desire. I understand that participation in this project
will not necessarily benefit me directly, but that information gained
from the project may someday benefit others.

                                        Date _____

                                   Signature _____

Check one: _____ Self

              _____ Parent

              _____ Guardian

Form A-5

Appendix B

REPRESENTATIVE REGULATIONS GOVERNING THE USE OF HUMAN SUBJECTS

NUREMBERG CODE (1946)*

Note: The Nuremberg Code, which was one of the first attempts to regulate human experimentation, consists of ten points that delimit permissible experimentation on human subjects. It was motivated by abuses in such experimentation that occurred in Nazi Germany during World War II.

1. The voluntary consent of the human subject is absolutely essential. This means that the person involved should have legal capacity to give consent; should be so situated as to be able to exercise free power of choice, without the intervention of any element of force, fraud, deceit, duress, over-reaching, or other ulterior form of constraint or coercion, and should have sufficient knowledge and comprehension of the elements of the subject matter involved as to enable him to make an understanding and enlightened decision. This latter element requires that before the acceptance of an affirmative decision by the experimental subject there should be made known to him the nature, duration, and purpose of the experiment; the method and means by which it is to be conducted, all inconveniences and hazards reasonably to be expected; and the effects upon his health or person which may possibly come from his participation in the experiment.

   The duty and responsibility for ascertaining the quality of the consent rests upon each individual who initiates, directs or engages in the experiment. It is a personal duty and responsibility which may not be delegated to another with impunity.

2. The experiment should be such as to yield fruitful results for the good of society, unprocurable by other methods or means of study, and not random and unnecessary in nature.

3. The experiment should be so designed and based on the results of animal experimentation and a knowledge of the natural history of the disease or other problem under study that the anticipated results will justify the performance of the experiment.

4. The experiment should be so conducted as to avoid all unnecessary physical and mental suffering and injury.

5. No experiment should be conducted where there is an *a priori* reason to believe that death or disabling injury will occur; except, perhaps, in those experiments where the experimental physicians also serve as subjects.

6. The degree of risk to be taken should never exceed that determined by the humanitarian importance of the problem to be solved by the experiment.

---

*Reprinted from "Permissible medical experiments" in *Trials of War Criminals before the Nuremberg Military Tribunals under Control Council Law No. 10: Nuremberg 1946 to April 1949*. Washington, D.C.: U.S. Government Printing Office (no date).

215

7. Proper preparations should be made and adequate facilities provided to protect the experimental subject against even remote possibilities of injury, disability, or death.
8. The experiment should be conducted only by scientifically qualified persons. The highest degree of skill and care should be required through all stages of the experiment of those who conduct or engage in the experiment.
9. During the course of the experiment the human subject should be at liberty to bring the experiment to an end if he has reached the physical or mental state where continuation of the experiment seems to him to be impossible.
10. During the course of the experiment the scientist in charge must be prepared to terminate the experiment at any stage, if he has probable cause to believe, in the exercise of the good faith, superior skill and careful judgment required of him that a continuation of the experiment is likely to result in injury, disability, or death of the experimental subject.

DECLARATION OF HELSINKI (1964)*

Note: This document has replaced the Nuremberg Code to some extent. The recommendations contained in it for conducting experiments using human subjects have been adopted by the World Medical Association. It represents one of the first attempts by the international scientific community to regulate human experimentation. Though its emphasis is medical, most of the recommendations are applicable to research in speech-language pathology and audiology. You may wish to substitute the word "clinician" for "doctor" while reading it. A somewhat expanded version of this code was adopted by the World Medical Association in 1975.

Introduction

It is the mission of the doctor to safeguard the health of the people. His knowledge and conscience are dedicated to the fulfillment of this mission. . . .

Because it is essential that the results of laboratory experiments be applied to human beings to further scientific knowledge and to help suffering humanity, the World Medical Association has prepared the following recommendations as a guide to each doctor in clinical research. It must be stressed that the standards as drafted are only a guide to physicians all over the world. Doctors are not relieved from criminal, civil and ethical responsibilities under the laws of their own countries.

In the field of clinical research a fundamental distinction must be recognized between clinical research in which the aim is essentially therapeutic for a patient, and the clinical research, the essential object of which is purely scientific and without therapeutic value to the person subjected to the research.

I. Basic Principles

1. Clinical research must conform to the moral and scientific principles that justify medical research and should be based on laboratory and animal experiments or other scientifically established facts.
2. Clinical research should be conducted only by scientifically qualified persons and under the supervision of a qualified medical man.

---

*Reprinted with permission of *The World Medical Journal.*

3. Clinical research cannot legitimately be carried out unless the importance of the objective is in proportion to the inherent risk to the subject.
4. Every clinical research project should be preceded by careful assessment of inherent risks in comparison to foreseeable benefits to the subject or to others.
5. Special caution should be exercised by the doctor in performing clinical research in which the personality of the subject is liable to be altered by drugs or experimental procedure.

II. Clinical Research Combined with Professional Care

1. In the treatment of the sick person, the doctor must be free to use a new therapeutic measure, if in his judgment it offers hope of saving life, reestablishing health, or alleviating suffering.
   If at all possible, consistent with patient psychology, the doctor should obtain the patient's freely given consent after the patient has been given a full explanation. In case of legal incapacity, consent should also be procured from the legal guardian; in the case of physical incapacity the permission of the legal guardian replaces that of the patient.
2. The doctor can combine clinical research with professional care, the objective being the acquisition of new medical knowledge, only to the extent that clinical research is justified by its therapeutic value for the patient.

III. Non-Therapeutic Clinical Research

1. In the purely scientific application of clinical research carried out on a human being, it is the duty of the doctor to remain the protector of the life and health of that person on whom clinical research is being carried out.
2. The nature, the purpose and the risk of clinical research must be explained to the subject by the doctor.
3a. Clinical research on a human being cannot be undertaken without his free consent after he has been informed; if he is legally incompetent, the consent of the legal guardian should be procured.
3b. The subject of clinical research should be in such a mental, physical and legal state as to be able to exercise fully his power of choice.
3c. Consent should, as a rule, be obtained in writing. However, the responsibility for clinical research always remains with the research worker; it never falls on the subject even after consent is obtained.
4a. The investigator must respect the right of each individual to safeguard his personal integrity, especially if the subject is in a dependent relationship to the investigator.
4b. At any time during the course of clinical research the subject or his guardian should be free to withdraw permission for research to be continued.

The investigator or the investigating team should discontinue the research if in his or their judgment, it may, if continued, be harmful to the individual.

Appendix C

SELECTED FEDERAL LEGISLATION RELEVANT TO SPEECH–LANGUAGE PATHOLOGISTS AND AUDIOLOGISTS

Americans with Disabilities Act of 1990 (P.L. 101-336). This act provides persons with disabilities the same protections against discrimination in the private sector that currently apply to minorities, women, and elderly persons. Persons with communicative impairments are covered by the act. For information about specific implications of the Act for such persons see Fox-Grimm (1991), ASHA work on ADA continues (1991), and Hurray for ADA! (1990).

Assistive Technology for Individuals with Disabilities Act (P.L. 100-407). This act provides support for the development of assistive technology devices and services, including that for augmentative communication.

Communication Act of 1934 (47 USCA 151). This act established the Federal Communications Commission, which has been concerned with the telecommunication needs of the deaf, hard-of-hearing, and speech impaired (including the establishment of TT [formerly TDD] and telecommunication relay services—see FCC broadens focus of telecommunications to include all persons with communication impairments, 1991).

Consumer Product Warranties (15 USCA 2301, Commerce and Trade). This act established rules governing the contents of warranties. It is relevant to speech-language pathologists and audiologists in their role as dispensers of products such as hearing aids and augmentative communication devices.

Developmental Disabilities Assistance and Bill of Rights (P.L. 101-496). This act assures that every person with a developmental disability has the opportunity for independence, productivity, and integration in to the community.

Education of All Handicapped Children Act (P.L. 94-142). This act was intended to assure that all handicapped children have available to them a free appropriate public education, including special education and related services, in the least restrictive environment (see Huffman, 1991). It has had a profound impact on the programming and delivery of speech, language, and hearing services in the public schools.

Education of the Handicapped Act Amendments of 1983 (P.L. 98-199). This amendment modified the definition of handicapped children in P.L. 94-142 to include "language impaired" after "hard of hearing, deaf, speech."

Education of the Handicapped Act Amendments of 1986 (P.L. 99-457). Title 1 of this act extends mandatory public school services to three- and four-year-old children with handicaps and provides incentives to states to offer services to infants and toddlers who are handicapped and at-risk and their families. It has profoundly affected the populations that speech-language pathologists and audiologists, particularly those employed by public schools, treat (see Crais & Leonard, 1990; Domico, 1989; Houle & Hamilton, 1991).

Federal Food, Drug, and Cosmetic Act (21 USCA 301). This act was intended to protect consumers from abuse and harm caused by the introduction, adulteration, or misbranding of any food, drug, *device*, or cosmetic in interstate commerce. Both hearing aids and augmentative communication devices are classified as "devices" under this act.

Federal Trade Commission: Promotion of Export Trade and Prevention of Unfair Methods of Competition (15 USCA 41, Commerce and Trade). This act created the Federal Trade Commission, which has attempted to alleviate anticompetitive practices in the hearing aid industry.

Hospital, Nursing Home, Domiciliary, and Medical Care (38 USCA 601, Veterans' Benefits). This act was intended to define eligibility for veterans to receive health-related services in Veterans' Administration and private facilities. The services covered by the act include those provided by speech-language pathologists and audiologists.

Individuals with Disabilities Education Act (IDEA) (P.L. 101-479). This act gives funding authority for the development of assistive technology and educational media and materials for youngsters with disabilities (see Support of assistive technology, 1991). The assistive technology covered includes that for augmentative communication.

Medical Devices Amendment (21 USCA 321). This act was intended to regulate the safety and efficacy of medical devices, including diagnostic and rehabilitative audiometric instrumentation.

National Deafness and Other Communication Disorders Act of 1988 (P.L. 100-553). This act established the National Institute on Deafness and Other Communication Disorders (NIDCD) as one of the 13 institutes of the National Institutes of Health (NIH) (see Snow, 1991).

Occupational Safety and Health Amendments of 1970 (P.L. 91-596). This act was intended to assure that all working men and women would have a "safe and healthful" work environment, one aspect of which would be an acceptable environmental noise level.

Rehabilitation Act of 1973 (P.L. 93-112). This act was intended to lessen discriminatory practices against handicapped persons. Section 504 states that "No otherwise qualified handicapped individual in the United States . . . shall, solely by reason of his handicap, be excluded from participation in, be denied the benefit of, or be subjected to discrimination under any program or activity receiving Federal financial assistance."

Sherman Antitrust Act (15 USCA 1, Commerce & Trade). This act was intended to prevent corporations and associations from engaging in restraint of trade. It has influenced ASHA's ethical guidelines for dispensing products (e.g., hearing aids) to persons with communicative disorders (see *Asha,* June 1978).

Social Security Act (42 USCA 301). This act funds several programs, including Medicare, that will pay for some speech, language, and hearing services for several subgroups of the communicatively handicapped population. Those eligible include some crippled children and aged persons. For further information about Medicare coverage of speech, language, and hearing services see Caniglia (1991), How to appeal Medicare denials (1990), Medicare documentation (1990), Medicare speech-language pathology medical review edits (1991), and White (1989).

Tax Reform Act of 1986 (TRA 86). This act does away with some tax advantages of setting up a business as a corporation. As such, the question of whether to incorporate a communication disorders private practice must be examined in a new light (see Hoops & Sliwoski, 1988).

Television Decoder Circuitry Act (P.L. 101-431). This act requires new television sets with screens thirteen inches or larger to have built-in decoder circuitry to display close-captioned television programming (see Captions: Getting the word out, 1990).

Voting Accessibility for the Elderly and Handicapped Act (P.L. 98-435). This act requires that voting and registration sites be accessible to handicapped and elderly voters, registration and voting information be obtainable using a TDD (TT), and printed instructions be available for the hearing impaired.

Appendix D

SELECTED ETHICAL CODES OF THE AMERICAN SPEECH-LANGUAGE-HEARING ASSOCIATION 1930–1991

PRINCIPLES OF ETHICS* (of the American Society for the Study of Disorders of Speech) (1930)

The Society proposes the following principles of ethics as an advisory instrument for the selection of new members, and for the professional guidance of present members.

Section I — Duties of Members to the Society. Members shall regard it as their duty and privilege to uphold the dignity and honor of the Society, to promote its interests and the welfare of its members, and to extend its sphere of usefulness whenever and wherever possible. They shall strive for the preservation and integrity of the Society through the practice of high personal standards of excellence in the pursuit of speech correction work, and shall seek to inspire in the public generally an impression of their dependability, culture, knowledge of techniques, and breadth of vision.

Section II — Secrecy. The obligation of secrecy so far as revelation of confidences of speech patients is concerned shall be regarded as a duty of members. Secrecy regarding methods and techniques, however, is opposed to the best interests of the Society; therefore each member shall attempt to extend the benefits of new methods, techniques, practical results, and experimental evidence to every member of the Society.

Section III — Unethical Practices. It shall be considered unethical:

1. To guarantee to cure any disorder of speech.
2. To offer in advance to refund any part of a person's tuition if his disorder of speech is not arrested.
3. To make "rash promises," difficult of fulfillment, in order to secure pupils or patients.
4. To employ blatant or untruthful methods of self-advertising.
5. To advertise to correct disorders of speech entirely by correspondence.
6. To seek self-advancement by attacking the work of other members of the Society in such a way as might injure their standing and reputation. Reproaches or criticisms should be sympathetically discussed with the member involved.

---

*This statement of ethical principles was quoted from Paden, 1970, pp. 74–75.

7. For persons who do not hold a medical degree to attempt to deal exclusively with speech patients requiring medical treatment without the advice or the authority of a physician.
8. To extend the time of treatment beyond the time when one should recognize his inability to effect further improvement.
9. To charge exorbitant fees for treatment.

CODE OF ETHICS OF THE AMERICAN SPEECH AND HEARING ASSOCIATION (1951)*

Section 1. Ethical Responsibilities of Members and Associates

The American Speech and Hearing Association is composed of persons having varying interests and professional duties, but certain broad ethical principles apply to the entire membership. The application of these principles to individual cases will depend on the particular circumstances of the professional duties and status of the persons involved.

It is convenient to divide the ethical responsibilities of persons in clinical professions into (1) those duties arising out of the relation between the professional worker and the person who seeks his assistance; (2) duties owed to other professional workers; and (3) obligations to society. These classifications are arbitrary, for actually the duties and responsibilities of the professional worker are indivisible. Any one of these ethical duties clearly implies the other two.

A. The most frequent professional relationship involving Members of ASHA is that of therapist to patient. The ethical responsibilities of this relationship demand that the welfare of the patient be considered paramount. Accordingly, the therapist must possess suitable qualifications for engaging in clinical work. Measures of such qualifications are provided by the Association's program for certification of the clinical competence of Members. The therapist must use every resource available, including referral to other specialists as needed, to effect as great improvement as possible in the shortest time consistent with good professional practice. Every precaution must be taken against causing any sort of injury to the patient. These general principles are understood and accepted by the profession and the public alike. Their application is the daily task of every professional clinical worker.

Another frequent professional relationship of ASHA Members and Associates is that of teacher to student. The broad ethical responsibilities of the teacher who is a Member or Associate of ASHA are in no way different from those of any other teacher, and no special statement of ethical requirements is in order.

B. The duties owed by Members and Associates to other professional workers are many. They should disseminate results of research and developments in speech and hearing therapy. They should avoid personal controversy, but should seek the freest professional discussion of all theoretical and practical issues. They should establish

---

*Reprinted from *Journal of Speech and Hearing Disorders*, 1952, pp. 255–256.

harmonious relationships with members of other professions, and should especially endeavor to inform them concerning the services that can be rendered by speech and hearing therapists. They should strive to promote the status of ASHA, of the professions of speech and hearing therapy, and of all therapy for and research concerning handicapping conditions.

C. The duties owed to society include first all the obligations of good citizenship which devolve upon members of human society. As persons with special training, ASHA Members and Associates have additional special responsibilities. They should help in the education of the public regarding speech and hearing problems and other matters lying within their professional competence. They should seek to provide and expand services to persons with speech and hearing handicaps, and assist in establishing high professional standards for such programs.

Section 2. Unethical practices.

A. It shall be considered unethical:

1. To guarantee the results of any speech or hearing consultative or therapeutic procedure. Any guarantee of any sort, express or implied, oral or written, is contrary to professional ethics. A therapist may always make a reasonable statement of prognosis, but a 'cure' or other specific favorable outcome is dependent upon many factors outside the therapist's control. Hence any warranty is deceptive and unethical.

2. To employ blatant or sensational advertising. The only form of advertising permissible is the so-called 'business card,' consisting of the name of the person or institution, the type of therapy offered, office hours, address, and telephone number. The words 'type of therapy' refer to such phrases as 'Speech Therapy,' 'Speech and Hearing Therapy,' 'Disorders of Speech,' and similar phrases. Members not holding clinical certification are expressly forbidden to use the name of the Association in advertising or any other professional promotion.

3. To diagnose or treat speech or hearing defects by correspondence. This does not preclude correspondence follow-up of patients previously seen personally.

4. To violate the patient's confidence by revealing any information obtained from or about him without his express permission. Case records must not be used in teaching in such a way as to permit identification of their subjects.

5. To write or say anything which may discredit professional colleagues or members of allied professions other than that based on adequate and objective evaluation of their work.

6. To exploit patients (a) by accepting for treatment patients whose defects cannot reasonably be expected to improve under therapy offered; (b) by continuing therapy unnecessarily; (c) by charging exorbitant fees.

7. To deal with speech patients requiring medical treatment without the advice of a physician.

8. For any student in training, whether on the undergraduate or the graduate level, to treat speech or hearing patients except as this treatment is given under competent supervision and as part of the training program. It will not, however, be considered unethical for a graduate student who holds a Basic Certificate to engage

in part-time speech or hearing therapy which is not part of the training program, provided that explicit approval of the director of such training program is secured in advance. A person holding a full-time clinical position and taking part-time graduate work is not, for the purpose of this Section, regarded as a student in training.

9. For any unqualified Member or Associate to treat speech or hearing patients, except under the supervision of one who is properly qualified.

10. To accept compensation from a dealer in prosthetic or other devices for recommending any particular device.

B. In addition to those which have been listed, other practices or actions might have an undesirable effect upon the patient, on relations with other professional personnel, or upon society, and would thus be unethical. It shall be the duty of the Committee on Ethical Practice to decide, in the light of all information it can collect, whether any specific act is in violation of the spirit of these Principles of Ethics.

CODE OF ETHICS OF THE AMERICAN SPEECH-LANGUAGE-HEARING ASSOCIATION 1991

(Revised January 1, 1991)

Preamble

The preservation of the highest standards of integrity and ethical principles is vital to the successful discharge of the professional responsibilities of all speech-language pathologists and audiologists. This Code of Ethics has been promulgated by the Association in an effort to stress the fundamental rules considered essential to this basic purpose. Any action that is in violation of the spirit and purpose of this Code shall be considered unethical. Failure to specify any particular responsibility or practice in this Code of Ethics should not be construed as denial of the existence of other responsibilities or practices.

The fundamental rules of ethical conduct are described in three categories: Principles of Ethics, Ethical Proscriptions, Matters of Professional Propriety.

1. *Principles of Ethics.* Five Principles serve as a basis for the ethical evaluation of professional conduct and form the underlying moral basis for the Code of Ethics. Individuals[1] subscribing to this Code shall observe these principles as affirmative obligations under all conditions of professional activity.

2. *Ethical Proscriptions.* Ethical Proscriptions are formal statements of prohibitions that are derived from the Principles of Ethics.

3. *Matters of Professional Propriety.* Matters of Professional Propriety represent guidelines of conduct designed to promote the public interest and thereby better inform the public and particularly the persons in need of speech-language pathology and audiology services as to the availability and the rules regarding the delivery of those services.

Principle of Ethics I

Individuals shall hold paramount the welfare of persons served professionally.

A. Individuals shall use every resource available, including referral to other specialists as needed, to provide the best service possible.

B. Individuals shall fully inform persons served of the nature and possible effects of these services.

C. Individuals shall fully inform subjects participating in research or teaching activities of the nature and possible effects of these activities.

D. Individuals' fees shall be commen-

---

[1] "Individuals" refers to all members of the American Speech-Language-Hearing Association and nonmembers who hold a Certificate of Clinical Competence from this Association.

surate with services rendered.

E. Individuals shall provide appropriate access to records of persons served professionally.

F. Individuals shall take all reasonable precautions to avoid injuring persons in the delivery of professional services.

G. Individuals shall evaluate services rendered and products dispensed to determine effectiveness.

Ethical Proscriptions

1. Individuals must not exploit persons in the delivery of professional services, including accepting persons for treatment when benefit cannot reasonably be expected or continuing treatment unnecessarily.

2. Individuals must not guarantee the results of any therapeutic procedures, directly or by implication. A reasonable statement of prognosis may be made, but caution must be exercised not to mislead persons served professionally to expect results that cannot be predicted from sound evidence.

3. Individuals must not use persons for teaching or research in a manner that constitutes invasion of privacy or fails to afford informed free choice to participate.

4. Individuals must not evaluate or treat speech, language or hearing disorders except in a professional relationship. They must not evaluate or treat solely by correspondence. This does not preclude follow-up correspondence with persons previously seen, nor providing them with general information of an educational nature.

5. Individuals must not reveal to unauthorized persons any professional or personal information obtained from the person served professionally, unless required by law or unless necessary to protect the welfare of the person or the community.

6. Individuals must not discriminate in the delivery of professional services on any basis that is unjustifiable or irrelevant to the need for and potential benefit from such services, such as race, sex, age, religion, national origin, sexual orientation, or handicapping condition.

7. Individuals must not charge for services not rendered.

Principle of Ethics II

Individuals shall maintain high standards of professional competence.

A. Individuals engaging in clinical practice or supervision thereof shall hold the appropriate Certificate(s) of Clinical Competence for the area(s) in which they are providing or supervising professional services.

B. Individuals shall continue their professional development throughout their careers.

C. Individuals shall identify competent, dependable referral sources for persons served professionally.

D. Individuals shall maintain adequate records of professional services rendered.

Ethical Proscriptions

1. Individuals must neither provide services nor supervision of services for which they have not been properly prepared, nor permit services to be provided by any of their staff who are not properly prepared.

2. Individuals must not provide clinical services by prescription of anyone who does not hold the Certificate of Clinical Competence.

3. Individuals must not delegate any service requiring the professional competence of a certified clinician to anyone unqualified.

4. Individuals must not offer clinical

services by supportive personnel, students or clinical fellows for whom they do not provide appropriate supervision and assume full responsibility.

5. Individuals must not require anyone under their supervision to engage in any practice that is a violation of the Code of Ethics.

Principle of Ethics III

Individuals' statements to persons served professionally and to the public shall provide accurate information about the nature and management of communicative disorders, and about the profession and services rendered by its practitioners.

Ethical Proscriptions

1. Individuals must not misrepresent their training or competence.

2. Individuals' public statements providing information about professional services and products must not contain representations or claims that are false, deceptive or misleading.

3. Individuals must not use professional or commercial affiliations in any way that would mislead or limit services to persons served professionally.

Matters of Professional Propriety

1. Individuals should announce services in a manner consonant with highest professional standards in the community.

Principle of Ethics IV

Individuals shall honor their responsibilities to the public, their profession, and their relationships with colleagues and members of allied professions.

Ethical Proscriptions

1. Individuals must not participate in activities that constitute a conflict of professional interest.

Matters of Professional Propriety

1. Individuals should seek to provide and expand services to persons with speech, language and hearing handicaps as well as to assist in establishing high professional standards for such programs.

2. Individuals should educate the public about speech, language and hearing processes, speech, language and hearing problems, and matters related to professional competence.

3. Individuals should strive to increase knowledge within the profession and share research with colleagues.

4. Individuals should establish harmonious relations with colleagues and members of other professions, and endeavor to inform members of related professions of services provided by speech-language pathologists and audiologists, as well as seek information from them.

5. Individuals should assign credit to those who have contributed to a publication in proportion to their contribution.

6. Individuals should not accept compensation for supervision or sponsorship from the clinical fellow being supervised or sponsored beyond reasonable reimbursement for direct expenses.

7. Individuals should present products they have developed to their colleagues in a manner consonant with highest professional standards.

Principle of Ethics V

Individuals shall uphold the dignity of the profession and freely accept the profession's self-imposed standards.
A. Individuals shall inform the Ethical Practice Board when they have reason to believe that a member or certificate holder may have violated the Code of Ethics.

B. Individuals shall cooperate fully with the Ethical Practice Board concerning matters of professional conduct related to this Code of Ethics.

Ethical Proscriptions

1. Individuals shall not engage in violations of the Principles of Ethics or in any attempt to circumvent any of them.

2. Individuals shall not engage in dishonesty, fraud, deceit, misrepresentation, or other forms of illegal conduct that adversely reflect on the profession or the individuals' fitness for membership in the profession.

GLOSSARY OF LEGAL TERMS*

Accreditation An approach used by a professional association to regulate the practice of an occupation through the establishment of standards for the curriculum and administration of programs that train new practitioners.

Administrative agency A rule-making organization created by a legislative or executive branch of government to develop, administer, and enforce the programs it has mandated in a specific subject matter area (e.g., education).

Administrative hearing A hearing conducted under the auspices of an administrative agency.

Administrative law The branch of law that deals with regulations promulgated by administrative agencies.

Advocate A person who does everything possible to insure that people receive the services that the law entitles them to receive.

Appellate courts Courts that review the decisions of trial courts when they are requested to do so.

Assault A tort resulting when someone's actions and/or words cause you to become apprehensive about being harmed by them.

Battery A tort resulting when someone intentionally touches you without your permission.

Bills Proposed laws considered by legislatures. If passed, they become statutes.

Breach of contract The failure of one or both parties to a contract to do what they agreed, or promised, to do.

Certification A voluntary mechanism by which a nongovernmental agency or association grants recognition to an individual who has met certain predetermined qualifications specified by that agency or association.

Civil law The branch of law concerned with relationships between private individuals, rather than between private individuals and society (which is the concern of criminal law).

Civil suit Litigation in which a court attempts to remedy a controversy between individuals or organizations.

Common law Legal precedent derived from court decisions.

Compensatory damages Damages intended to compensate the plaintiff for the injury he or she received from the defendant.

Complaint A document drafted by the attorney for the plaintiff in a lawsuit that

---

*Many of the terms relevant to law that were used in this book are briefly defined here. For definitions of other terms or for more complete definitions of those defined, consult the index.

indicates why the plaintiff believes he or she was legally wronged by the defendant and specifies the judicial remedy being sought.

Contract A promise or set of promises for breach of which the law gives a remedy, or the performance of which the law in some way recognizes as a duty.

Copyright The exclusive right to make and sell copies of an author's work for a limited period of time.

Corporation A business (e.g., private practice) that obtains its financing by selling stock, or shares of ownership; it is classified by the courts as a person.

Countersuit A lawsuit initiated against the plaintiff by the defendant. In a countersuit the defendant becomes the plaintiff and the plaintiff the defendant.

Criminal law The branch of law that deals with crimes, or acts against society.

Damages Money that the plaintiff is seeking from the defendant in a lawsuit to compensate for an "injury" that the plaintiff feels was done to him or her by the defendant.

Declaratory judgment A statement of clarification that a person seeks from a court regarding what the law is in a particular situation or the meaning of the law in that situation.

Defamation A tort that results from saying or writing something false and malicious about someone that injures their reputation. It includes both slander and libel.

Defendant The person sued by the plaintiff in a lawsuit.

Deposition A statement made under oath in writing, ordinarily prior to a trial.

Discovery An opportunity given to each party in a lawsuit to find out prior to the trial the sorts of evidence the other party has and is likely to use at the trial.

Ex post facto laws Laws that make a crime of an act that, when it was done, was not a crime.

Expert witness A witness who both evaluates and provides evidence in his or her area of expertise.

Felonies Crimes that are not classified as misdemeanors. They usually are punishable by relatively large fines, relatively long prison sentences, and in some extremely serious cases, death.

Fraud An intentional perversion of truth for the purpose of inducing another who relies on it to part with some valuable belonging or to surrender a legal right.

Functionalism A philosophy that suggests that the decision the courts are most likely to make in a particular situation can be regarded as the law in that situation.

Informed consent Consent given by a research subject or client that was not obtained by coercion and did not result from the person's failing to be fully informed about the risks involved.

Injunction An order issued by a court to a defendant to do some specific activity or to refrain from doing some specific activity.

Intentional torts Torts that result from acts that are intended to injure or harm others and/or are morally wrong.

Laws Rules that are intended to govern our interpersonal relationships; they place restrictions and obligations on our relations with others.

Libel Defamation tort resulting from false and malicious statements being communicated in written or printed form.

Licensure A legal mechanism by which a governmental agency authorizes persons who have met specified minimal standards of competency to engage in a given profession or occupation.

Licensure board A state administrative agency responsible for administering a licensure law.

Liquidated damages A specific amount of money specified in a contract that the party who breaches a contract agrees to pay to the other party in the contract.

Litigation A legal proceeding.

Lobbyist Any person who intentionally attempts to influence how legislators vote.

Malpractice Any type of negligent conduct by a professional that causes his or her patient (client) to be harmed either physically or emotionally.

Misdemeanors Relatively minor crimes that usually are punishable by relatively low fines and/or relatively short terms of imprisonment.

Natural law A philosophy suggesting that we have an obligation in our interpersonal relationships to do what is "right," "fair," "just," and "ethical."

Negligence torts Torts involving carelessness that injures or harms others (e.g., malpractice).

Nominal damages Small amounts of money that are awarded to plaintiffs when the wrong done to them did not result in an actual injury.

Partnership A business (e.g., private practice) owned by two or more persons.

Patent A grant made by the government to an inventor, conveying and securing to him or her the exclusive right to make, use, and sell the invention for a term of years.

Plaintiff The person (or group) who initiates a lawsuit (i.e., files a complaint).

Positive law A philosophy stating that the law is what legally constituted lawmakers say it is.

Pro se litigant A defendant or plaintiff in a lawsuit who acts as his or her own attorney.

Procedural laws Laws that specify how substantive laws are to be enforced.

Property law The branch of civil law concerned with rights of ownership.

Proprietorship A business (e.g., private practice) owned by a single person.

Punitive damages Damages awarded to the plaintiff in addition to compensatory damages; their purpose is to punish the defendant.

Realism A philosophy suggesting that the unconscious prejudices judges hold are likely to influence their court decisions.

Record An account of what has been done.

Reformation A type of remedy that can be ordered by a court when a contract does not accurately reflect the agreement between the parties because of error, fraud, or ambiguous language. It is an order to revise the contract.

Registration A form of certification administered by a governmental agency in which persons who have completed the training deemed necessary by the agency to function as practitioners in a particular field have their names listed in a register (file) that is maintained by the agency.

Restitution A type of remedy that can be ordered by a court if a plaintiff has been unjustly deprived of a right or property. Restitution may or may not involve money.

Slander Defamation tort resulting from false or malicious statements being communicated in oral form.

Stare decisis The tendency of judges to base their decisions on precedent, when precedent exists, and thus not decide what already has been decided.

Statute A law passed by a legislature.

Statute of limitations A statute that specifies how long a person has after an event has occurred to initiate a suit in relation to it. A plaintiff may not be awarded the remedy sought because he or she has waited too long to initiate a suit.

Subpoena An order issued by a court to turn over certain documents to it or to testify; it is issued when a person refuses to do so voluntarily.

Substantive laws Laws that create, define, and regulate duties and rights. Such laws tell us what we should and should not do.

Summons A document that directs a person to appear in court to answer a complaint.

Torts Injuries or wrongs to individuals resulting from the dangerous or unreasonable conduct of others, that do not arise from breaching a contract, for which courts will provide a remedy by awarding compensation.

Trial courts The first courts to try, consider, or become involved with any civil or criminal case. They are at the entrance level in the hierarchies of both state and federal court systems.

Utilitarianism A philosophy that suggests that legislatures (and other lawmakers) should attempt to promote the greatest good for the greatest number of persons by making appropriate laws.

REFERENCES

Actions of the Ethical Practice Board (1986). *Asha,* 28 (7), 51.

Actions of the Ethical Practice Board (1988). *Asha,* 30 (1), 59.

Actions of the Ethical Practice Board (1989a). *Asha,* 31 (9), 47.

Actions of the Ethical Practice Board (1989b). *Asha,* 31 (11), 59.

Actions of the Ethical Practice Board (1991a). *Asha,* 33 (1), 68.

Actions of the Ethical Practice Board (1991b). *Asha,* 33 (4), 70.

Actions of the Ethical Practice Board (1991c). *Asha,* 33 (8), 55.

ALTMAN, L., & MELCHER, L. (1983). Fraud in science. *British Medical Journal,* 286, 2003–2006.

ANNAS, G. J. (1975). *The Rights of Hospital Patients: The Basic ACLU Guide to a Hospital Patient's Rights.* New York: Avon Books.

ASHA–PAC: A visible influence (1988). *Asha,* 30 (9), 57.

ASHA–PAC wants effective leaders (1990). *Asha,* 32 (8), 33.

ASHA work on ADA continues (1991). *Governmental Affairs Review,* 12 (4), 8.

BAILAR, J. C. (1986). Science, statistics, and deception. *Annals of Internal Medicine,* 104, 259–260.

BANGS, J. L. (1970). Third party payment abuses. *Asha,* 12, 418.

BATTIN, R. R., & FOX, D. R. (Eds.) (1978). *Private Practice in Audiology and Speech Pathology.* New York: Grune & Stratton.

BEBOUT, M. (1986). The malpractice storm. *Hearing Journal,* 39 (2), 7–12.

BLACK, H. C. (1968). *Black's Law Dictionary* (Rev. 4th Ed.). St. Paul, Minn.: West Publishing.

BLOCK, E. (1975). *Voice Printing.* New York: David McKay.

BLOODSTEIN, O. (1988). Verification of stuttering in a suspected malingerer. *Journal of Fluency Disorders,* 13, 83–88.

BRIDGMAN, P. W. (1961). *The Logic of Modern Physics.* New York: Macmillan.

BRODY, B. A. (1978). Law and morality. In Warren T. Reich (Ed.), *Encyclopedia of Bioethics,* Volume 2. New York: Free Press.

BROWNE, J. T. (1991). May you live with "interesting" laws: Government regulation in the 1990s. *Asha,* 33 (6), 39–40.

BUTLER, K. G. (Ed.) (1986). *Prospering in Private Practice.* Rockville, Maryland: Aspin.

CANIGLIA, J. A. (1991). Information is of essence. *Asha,* 33 (8), 12–13.

CAPLAN, M. (1983). *Ralph Nadar Presents a Citizen's Guide to Lobbying.* New York: Norton.

Captions: Getting the word out (1990). *Asha,* 32 (6), 11.

CARNEY, P. J. (1991). Competence: An ethical decision. *Asha,* 33 (4), 7–8.

Casebook on Ethical Principles for Psychologists (1987). Washington, D.C.: American Psychological Association.

CHARLES, S. C., & KENNEDY, E. (1985). *Defendant.* New York: Free Press.

CHICKERING, R. B., & HARTMANM S. (1987). *How to Register a Copyright and Protect Your Creative Work.* New York: Charles Scribner's Sons.

CIUCCIO, J. (1990). Ethics, nostrums, and quackery. *Asha,* 33 (8), 38–39.

Code of Ethics of the American Speech-Language-Hearing Association (1991). *Asha,* 33 (3), 103–104.

Congressional Action Contact Network Handbook (1991). Rockville, Maryland: American Speech-Language-Hearing Association.

COOPER, E. B. (Summer, 1991). Standards and licensure in speech-language pathology and audiology. *Licensure Newsletter.*

CORBIN, A. L. (1952). *Corbin on Contracts.* St. Paul, Minnesota: West Publishing.

Council on Professional Standards (1991). Accreditation of professional services programs proposed standards revision. *Asha,* 33 (6), 49–52.

CRAIS, E. R., & LEONARD, C. R. (1990). PL 99-457: Are speech-language pathologists prepared for the challenge? *Asha,* 32 (4), 57–61.

CROLL, R. P. (1984). The noncontributing author: An issue of credit and responsibility. *Perspectives in Biology and Medicine,* 27, 401–407.

CUPPIES, B., & GOCHNAUER, M. (1985). The investigator's duty not to deceive. *IRB: A Review of Human Subjects Research,* 7 (5), 1–6.

DAVIS, K. C. (1977). *Administrative Law: Cases-Text-Problems.* St. Paul, Minn.: West Publishing.

DIBLE, D. M. (Ed.) (1978). *What Everybody Should Know About Patents, Trademarks, and Copyrights.* Fairfield, Calif.: Entrepreneur Press.

Digest of State Laws and Regulations for School Language, Speech, and Hearing Programs (1973). Rockville, Md.: American Speech-Language-Hearing Association.

DOMICO, W. D. (1989). The 1986 Education of the Handicapped Act and judicial decisions relating to the child who is hearing impaired. *Asha,* 31 (9), 91–95.

DOWLING, R. J. (1973). *ASHA Handbook for Congressional Action Contacts.* Rockville, Maryland: American Speech-Language-Hearing Association.

DOWNEY, M. (1979). Legal developments—Antitrust and sunset laws. *Asha,* 21, 7–11.

DOWNEY, M. (1980a). Conduct of the due process hearing. *Asha,* 22, 332–333.

DOWNEY, M. (1980b). Due process hearings and PL 94-142. *Asha,* 22, 255–257.

DUBOW, S. (1982). *Legal Rights of Hearing Impaired People.* Washington, D. C.: National Center for Law and the Deaf.

EDELSTEIN, L. (1943). The Hippocratic Oath: Text, translation, and interpretation. *Bulletin of the History of Medicine,* Supplement 1. Baltimore: Johns Hopkins University Press.

EPB interpretation of "Joint Committee Statement on Tongue Thrust" (1975). *Asha,* 17, 331.

Ethical practices board interpretations of principles governing the dispensing of products to persons with communicative disorders (1976). *Asha,* 18, 227–240.

Ethical Practice Board statement of practices and procedures (1991). *Asha,* 33 (3), 105–106.

FCC broadens focus of telecommunications to include all persons with communication impairments (1991). *Governmental Affairs Review,* 12 (5), 3.

Final regulations amending basic HSS policy for the protection of human research subjects (1981). *Federal Register,* 46, 8366–8392.

FEUER, W. W. (1990). *Medical Malpractice Law.* Irvine, Calif.: LawPrep Press.

FISHER, B. D. (1977). *Introduction to the Legal System* (2nd Ed.). St. Paul, Minn.: West Publishing.

FLETCHER, J. C., DOMMEL, JR., & COWELL, D. D. (1985). Consent to research with impaired human subjects. *IRB: A Review of Human Subjects Research,* 7 (6), 1–6.

FLOWER, R. M. (1986). Ethical concerns in private practice. In Katherine G. Butler (Ed.), *Prospering in Private Practice.* Rockville, Maryland: Aspin.

FOX, D. R. (1978). Forensic speech pathology. In R. Ray Battin & Donna R. Fox (Eds.), *Private Practice in Audiology and Speech Pathology.* New York: Grune & Stratton.

FOX–GRIMM, M. E. (1991). Americans With Disabilities Act: PL 101-336. *Asha,* 33 (6), 41–43, 45.

FREEDMAN, B. (1987). Scientific value and validity as ethical requirements for research: A proposed explication. *IRB: A Review of Human Subjects Research,* 9 (6), 7–10.

FREEDMAN, B. (1990). Placebo-controlled trials and the logic of clinical purpose. *IRB: A Review of Human Subjects Research,* 12 (6), 1–6.

FREUND, P. (Ed.) (1970). *Experimentation with Human Subjects.* New York: George Braziller.

FRIED, C. (1974). *Medical Experimentation: Personal Integrity and Social Policy.* New York: American Elsevier.

FRIEDENWALD, H. (1917). *Bulletin of the Johns Hopkins Hospital,* 28, 260–261.

GASS, R. S. (1978). Codes of the health-care professions. In Warren T. Reich (Ed.), *Encyclopedia of Bioethics,* Volume 4. New York: Free Press.

GIFIS, S. H. (1991). *Law Dictionary* (Third Edition). Woodbury, N. Y.: Barron's Educational Service.

Governmental regulation: A statement by the American Speech and Hearing Association (1969). *Asha,* 11, 39–43.

GREENWALD, R. A., RYAN, M. K., & MULVIHILL, J. E. (1982). *Human Subjects Research: A Handbook for Institutional Review Boards.* New York: Plenum Press.

GRILLIOT, H. J. (1979). *Introduction to Law and the Legal System* (2nd Ed.). Boston: Houghton Mifflin.

GRINNELL, F. (1990). Endings of clinical research protocols: Distinguishing therapy from research. *IRB: A Review of Human Subjects Research,* 12 (4), 1–3.

HARING, B. (1975). *Ethics of Manipulation.* New York: Seabury Press.

HAYT, E., HAYT, L. R., & GROESCHEL, A. H. (1972). *Law of Hospital, Physician, and Patient* (3rd Ed.). Berwyn, Ill.: Physicians' Record Company.

HEITMAN, F. D. (1980). State Licensure: The Profession of Speech Pathology and Audiology. Unpublished doctoral dissertation, University of Florida.

HILTGARTNER, S. (1990). Research fraud, misconduct, and the IRB. *IRB: A Review of Human Subjects Research*, 12 (1), 1–4.

HOEDEMAN, P. (1991). *Hitler or Hippocrates: Medical Experiments and Euthanasia in the Third Reich.* Sussex, England: The Book Guild.

HOLDER, A. R. (1989). Researchers and subpoenas: The troubling precedent of the Selikoff case. *IRB: A Review of Human Subjects Research*, 11 (6), 8–10.

HOOPS, H. R., & SLIWOSKI, L. (1988). The Tax Reform Act of 1986 and the private practice incorporation decision. *Asha*, 30 (1), 41–44.

HOULE, G. R., & HAMILTON, J. L. (1991). Public Law 99-457: A challenge to speech-language pathologists and audiologists. *Asha*, 33 (4), 51–54.

How to appeal Medicare denials (1990). *Asha*, 32 (12), 8–9.

HUFFMAN, N. P. (1991). Least restrictive environment. *Asha*, 33 (6), 43–45.

Hurray for ADA! (1990). *Asha*, 32 (9), 13.

Implementation procedures for the standards for the Certificate of Clinical Competence (1991). *Asha*, 33 (5), 47–53.

IMWINKELRIED, J. (1980). *Evidentiary Foundations.* New York: Bobbs-Merrill.

INTERNATIONAL AUSCHWITZ COMMITTEE (1986). *Nazi Medicine: Doctors, Victims, and Medicine in Auschwitz.* New York: Howard Fertig.

Issues in ethical practice—responsibilities concerning the honoring of a verbal or written contract (1958). *Journal of Speech and Hearing Disorders*, 23, 160–161.

Issues in ethics: Identification of members engaged in clinical practice without certification (1973). *Asha*, 15, 381.

Issues in ethics: Advertising of members' products (1974). *Asha*, 16, 44.

Issues in ethics: The bogus degree (1974). *Asha*, 16, 212.

Issues in ethics: CFY supervisors' responsibilities (1974). *Asha*, 16, 212.

Issues in ethics: Guidelines for telephone directories (1974). *Asha*, 16, 708–709.

Issues in ethics: Clinical practice by members in the area in which they are not certified (1977). *Asha*, 19, 343.

Issues in ethics: Public statements and general announcements: Guidelines and procedures (1977). *Asha*, 19, 423.

Issues in ethics: Gratuities (1978). *Asha*, 20, 311–312.

Issues in ethics: Fees for clinical services provided by students (1978). *Asha*, 20, 427.

Issues in ethics: Ethical practice inquiries: State versus ASHA decision differences (1978). *Asha*, 20, 505–506.

Issues in ethics: ASHA policy re. supportive personnel (1979). *Asha*, 21, 419.

Issues in ethics: CFY supervisors' responsibilities (1980a). *Asha*, 22, 273–274.

Issues in Ethics: Drawing cases for private practice from primary place of employment (1980b). *Asha* 22, 939.

Issues in ethics: Public announcements and public statements (1981). *Asha*, 23, 107.

Issues in Ethics: Ethics in research and professional practice (1982). *Asha*, 24, 1029–1031.

Issues in Ethics: Clinical practice by certificate holders in areas in which they are not certified (1986). *Asha*, 28 (4), 58.

Issues in Ethics: Use of graduate degrees by members and/or certificate holders (1987). *Asha*, 29 (6), 42.

Issues in Ethics: Competition (1989a). *Asha,* 31 (9), 45.

Issues in Ethics: Prescription (1989b). *Asha,* 31 (9), 45.

Issues in Ethics: Supervision of student clinicians (1991). *Asha,* 33 (10), 53.

JEANS, J. W. (1975). *Trial Advocacy.* St. Paul, Minn.: West Publishing.

JOHNSON, W. (1946). *People in Quandaries.* New York: Harper & Row.

JONES, J. H. (1981). *Bad Blood: The Tuskegee Syphilis Experiment.* New York: Free Press.

KATES, B., MCNAUGHTON, S., & SILVERMAN, H. (no date). *Handbook of Blissymbolics for Instructors, Users, Parents, and Administrators.* Toronto: Blissymbolics Communication Institute.

KATZ, J., BASIL, R. A., & SMITH, J. M. (1963). A staggered spondaic test for detecting central auditory lesions. *Annals of Otology, Rhinology, and Laryngology,* 72, 908–918.

KOENIGSKNECHT, R. A. (1990a). Ethics: For goodness sake. *Asha,* 32 (9), 7–8.

KOENIGSKNECHT, R. A. (1990b). Go in the name of the law. *Asha,* 32 (11), 7–8.

KOENIGSKNECHT, R. A. (1990c). Learn from our consumers. *Asha,* 32 (6), 33–34.

KONOLD, D. (1978). Codes of medical ethics: I. History. In Warren T. Reich (Ed.), *Encyclopedia of Bioethics,* Volume 1. New York: Free Press.

KOOPER, R., & SULLIVAN, C. A. (1986). Professional liability: Management and prevention. In Katherine G. Butler (Ed.), *Prospering in Private Practice.* Rockville, Maryland: Aspin.

KORZYBSKI, A. (1933). *Science and Sanity.* Lakeville, Conn.: Institute of General Semantics.

KOZAK, E. (1990). *Every Writer's Guide to Copyright and Publishing Law.* New York: Henry Holt.

KRAMER, M. B., & ARMBRUSTER, J. M. (Eds.) (1982). *Forensic Audiology.* Baltimore: University Park Press.

LADIMER, I. (1970). Protection and compensation for injury in human studies. In Paul A. Freund (Ed.), *Experimentation with Human Subjects.* New York: George Braziller.

LC amends Code of Ethics (1990). *Asha,* 32 (4), 10.

LEHRHOFF, I., & KORASHEC, S. (no date). *Speech and Language Procedure Manual.* Beverly Hills, Calif.: Irwin Lehrhoff and Associates.

LEVINE, A. H., & CARY, E. (1977). *The Rights of Students: The Basic ACLU Guide to a Student's Rights.* New York: Avon Books.

LEVINE, L. B. (1978). Institutional licensure versus individual licensure. *Journal of Allied Health,* 7, 109–114.

LEVINE, R. J. (1983). Research involving children: An interpretation of the new regulations. *IRB: A Review of Human Subjects Research,* 5 (4), 1–5.

LEVINE, R. J. (1986). *Ethics and Regulation of Clinical Research* (Second Edition). Baltimore-Munich: Urban & Schwarzenberg.

Liability lawsuits present danger to qualified professionals, says official (1985). *Asha,* 27 (6), 9–10.

LOWE, R. G. (1988). Are audiologists guilty of malpractice if they do not recommend binaural amplification? *Asha,* 30 (11), 39–40.

LYNCH, C. (1986). Harm to the public: Is it real? *Asha,* 28 (6), 25–31.

LYNCH, C. (1988). 1988 policy issues and activities in the states. *Asha,* 30 (12), 45–48.

LYNCH, C. (1990). Characteristics of state licensure laws. *Asha,* 32 (11), 47–55.

LYNCH, C., & DUBINSKE, S. (1986). Licensure in speech-language pathology and audiology: The questions/the answers. *Asha,* 28 (6), 33–36.

LUM, J. (1979). Reference groups and professional socialization. In Margaret Hardy & Mary E. Conway (Eds.), *Role Theory: Prospectives for Health Professionals.* Englewood Cliffs, N. J.: Prentice-Hall.

MACHOVEC, F. (1987). *The Expert Witness Survival Manual.* Springfield, Illinois: Charles C Thomas.

MACKLIN, R. (1989). The paradoxical case of payment as benefit to research subjects. *IRB: A Review of Human Subjects Research,* 6 (11), 1–3.

MAULET, T. A. (1980). *Fundamentals of Trial Techniques.* New York: Little, Brown.

MCDOWELL, B. (1991). *Ethical Conduct and the Professional Dilemma: Choosing Between Service and Success.* New York: Quorum Books.

MCLARTY, J. W. (1987). How many subjects are required for a study? *IRB: A Review of Human Subjects Research,* 9 (5), 1–3.

Medicare documentation (1990). *Asha,* 32 (8), 12–13.

Medicare speech-language pathology medical review edits (1991). *Asha,* 33 (9), 57–60.

MESLIN, E. M. (1990). Protecting human subjects from harm through improved risk judgments. *IRB: A Review of Human Subjects Research,* 12 (1), 7–10.

METZ, D. E., & FOLKINS, J. W. (1985). Protection of human subjects in speech and hearing research. *Asha,* 27 (3), 25–29.

MEYERS, L. J. (1968). *The Law and the Deaf.* Washington, D. C.: Vocational Rehabilitation Administration.

MILLER, T. D. (1983). Professional Liability in Speech-Language Pathology and Audiology: Unprofessional Conduct and Unethical Practice. Unpublished doctoral dissertation, State University of New York at Buffalo.

MILLER, T. D., & LUBINSKI, R. (1986). Professional liability in speech-language pathology and audiology. *Asha,* 28 (6), 45–47.

MOENSSENS, A. A. (1973). *Scientific Evidence in Criminal Cases.* Mineola, N. Y.: Foundation Press.

MORRIS, W. O. (1984). *Revocation of Professional Licenses by Governmental Agencies.* Charlottesville, Virginia: The Michie Company.

National forum on consumer rights (1990). *Asha,* 32 (6), 35–39.

NEWTON, L. H. (1984). Agreement to participate in research: Is that a promise? *IRB: A Review of Human Subjects Research,* 6 (2), 7–9.

NICHOLAS, T. (1977). *How to Form Your Own Corporation Without a Lawyer for Under $50.00.* Wilmington, Dela.: Enterprise Publishing.

Non-speech communication: A position paper (1980). *Asha,* 22, 267–272.

NORMAN, M. C. (1986). National Council of State Boards of Examiners for Speech-Language Pathology and Audiology. *Asha,* 28 (6), 23.

Ohio Federal District Court allows ASHA to file as *Amicus Curiae* (1991). *Asha,* 33 (8), 9.

OSTBERG, K. (1990). *Using a Lawyer . . . And What to Do If Things Go Wrong: A Step-By-Step Guide.* New York: Random House.

O'TOOLE, T. J. (1974). The speech clinician and child abuse. *Language, Speech, and Hearing Services in Schools,* 5, 103–106.

OULAHAN, C. (1978). The legal implications of evaluation and accreditation. *Journal of Law and Education,* 7, 193–238.

PADEN, E. P. (1970). *A History of the American Speech and Hearing Association, 1925-1958.* Rockville, Md.: American Speech-Language-Hearing Association.

PORCH, B. E. (1967). *Porch Index of Communicative Ability.* Palo Alto, Calif.: Consulting Psychologists Press.

Perspectives on licensure (1986). *Asha,* 28 (6), 19–23.

Position statement on nonspeech communication (1981). *Asha,* 23, 577–581.

PROSSER, W. L. (1971). *Law of Torts* (4th Ed.). St. Paul, Minn.: West Publishing.

PURTILO, R. B., & CASSEL, C. K. (1981). *Ethical Dimensions in the Health Professions.* Philadelphia: W. B. Saunders.

RADA, R. T., PORCH, B., & KELLNER, R. (1975). Aphasia and expert medical witness. *American Academy of Psychiatry and the Law Bulletin,* 3, 231–237.

RADIL–WEISS, T. (1983). Men in extreme conditions: Some medical and psychological aspects of the Auschwitz concentration camp. *Psychiatry,* 46, 259–268.

REECE, R. D., & SIEGAL, H. A. (1986). *Studying People: A Primer in the Ethics of Social Research.* Macon, Georgia: Mercer University Press.

REICH, W. T. (Ed.) (1978). *Encyclopedia of Bioethics,* Volume 4. New York: Free Press.

Restatement of the Law: Contracts. St. Paul, Minn.: American Law Institute. Copyright 1973 by the American Law Institute. All quotations reprinted with permission of the American Law Institute.

Restatement of the Law: Torts (2nd Ed.). St. Paul, Minn.: American Law Institute. Copyright 1979 by the American Law Institute. All quotations reprinted with permission of the American Law Institute.

ROEMER, R. (1974). Trends in licensure, certification, and accreditation: Implications for health-manpower education in the future. *Journal of Allied Health,* 3, 26–33.

ROMBAUER, M. D. (1978). *Legal Problem Solving.* St. Paul, Minn.: West Publishing.

ROSNER, R., & WEINSTOCK, R. (1990). *Ethical Practice in Psychiatry and the Law.* New York: Plenem Press.

ROTTENBERG, S. (1968). Licensing, occupational. In D. L. Sills (Ed.), *International Encyclopedia of the Social Sciences.* Volume 9. New York: Macmillan and Free Press, 283–285.

ROWLAND, R. C. (1988). Malpractice in audiology and speech-language pathology. *Asha,* 30 (1), 45–48.

SANBAR, S. S. (May 1977). The expert witness. Paper presented at the American Academy of Private Practice in Speech Pathology and Audiology Conference on Legal Considerations, Oklahoma City.

SCHRIFTGIESSER, K. (1951). *The Lobbyists.* Boston: Little, Brown.

SCHULER, H. (1982). *Ethical Problems in Psychological Research.* New York: Academic Press.

SEELMAN, K. D. (February, 1991). The ABS's of the Relay Service. *SHHH Journal,* pp. 4–6.

SHAPIRO, D. L. (1984). *Psychological Evaluation and Expert Testimony: A Practical Guide to Forensic Work.* New York: Van Nostrand Reinhold.

SHIRKEY, E. A. (1987). Forensic verification of stuttering. *Journal of Fluency Disorders,* 12, 197–203.

SIEBER, J. E. (1989). Sharing scientific data I: New problems for IRBs. *IRB: A Review of Human Subjects Research,* 11 (6), 4–7.

SILVERMAN, F. H. (1989). *Communication for the Speechless* (2nd Ed.). Englewood Cliffs, N. J.: Prentice Hall.

SILVERMAN, F. H. (1993). *Research Design and Evaluation in Speech-Language Pathology and Audiology* (3rd Ed.). Englewood Cliffs, N. J.: Prentice Hall.

SNOW, JR., J. B. (1991). A new institute: A promising future of research. *Asha,* 33 (9), 33–34.

Standards for accreditation of educational programs (1990). *Asha,* 32 (6), 93–94, 100.

Standards for federal funding (1972). *Asha,* 14, 546–550.

STEWART, W. W., & FEDER, N. (1987). The integrity of the scientific literature. *Nature,* 325, 207–214.

STRONG, W. S. (1990). *The Copyright Book: A Practical Guide* (Third Edition). Cambridge, Mass.: MIT Press.

Study of Accreditation of Selected Health Education Programs — Commission Report (1973). Washington, D. C.: Department of Health, Education, & Welfare.

Support of assistive technology (1991). *Governmental Affairs Review,* 12 (4), 6.

Survey of sunset laws (1991). *Governmental Affairs Review,* 12 (3), 15.

TAUB, H. A. (1986). Comprehension of informed consent for research: Issues and directions for future study. *IRB: A Review of Human Subjects Research,* 8 (6), 7–10.

THOMPSON, R. A. (1990). Behavioral research involving children: A developmental perspective on risk. *IRB: A Review of Human Subjects Research,* 12 (2), 1–6.

TUCKER, B. P., & GOLDSTEIN, B. A. (1991). *Legal Rights of Persons with Disabilities.* Horsham, PA: LRP Publications.

VEATCH, R. M. (1987). *The Patient as Partner: A Theory of Human-Experimentation Ethics.* Bloomington: Indiana University Press.

VAN RIPER, C. (1973). *The Treatment of Stuttering.* Englewood Cliffs, N. J.: Prentice Hall.

The Washington connection: *Asha* interviews Morgan Downey (1981). *Asha,* 23, 480–483.

The Washington Lobby (1971). Washington, D. C.: Congressional Quarterly.

WEBSTER, R. A. (1974). A behavioral analysis of stuttering: Treatment and theory. In K. Calhoun et al. (Eds.), *Innovative Treatment Methods in Psychopathology.* New York: John Wiley.

WEIL, V., & HOLLANDER, R. (1990). Sharing scientific data II: Normative issues. *IRB: A Review of Human Subjects Research,* 12 (2), 7–8.

WEITHORN, L. A. (1983). Children's capacities to decide about participation in research. *IRB: A Review of Human Subjects Research,* 5 (2), 1–5.

WENKE, R. A. (1989). *The Art of Selecting a Jury* (2nd Ed.). Springfield, Illinois: Charles C Thomas.

WHITE, S. C. (1986). Licensure and third party reimbursement. *Asha,* 28 (6), 36.

WHITE, S. C. (1989). Medicare and nursing home services. *Asha,* 31 (4), 75, 59.

WISHMAN, S. (1986). *Anatomy of a Jury.* New York: Times Books.

WOLF, K. E., POWELL, R. H., & MONTGOMERY, J. K. (1989). Involvement in the legislative process through the state association. *Asha,* 31 (4), 37–38, 78.

WOLPE, B. C. (1990). *Lobbying Congress: How the System Works.* Washington, D. C.: Congressional Quarterly.

WOOD, M. L. (1986). *Private Practice in Communication Disorders.* Boston: Little, Brown.

WOODY, R. H. (1986). Legal issues for private practitioners in speech-language pathology and audiology. In Katherine G. Butler (Ed.), *Prospering in Private Practice.* Rockville, Maryland: Aspin.

You and the Law (2nd Ed.) (1977). Pleasantville, N. Y.: Reader's Digest Association.

INDEX

241

DATE DUE

MAR 27 '95			